MRCP Part 1
Self-Assessment

Medical Masterclass questions and explanatory answers

EDITED BY

John D Firth DM FRCP

Consultant Physician and Nephrologist
Addenbrooke's Hospital
Cambridge

FOREWORD BY

Professor Ian Gilmore MD PRCP

President
Royal College of Physicians

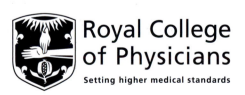

Royal College
of Physicians
Setting higher medical standards

Radcliffe Publishing
Oxford • New York

Radcliffe Publishing Ltd
18 Marcham Road
Abingdon
Oxon OX14 1AA
United Kingdom

www.radcliffe-oxford.com
Electronic catalogue and worldwide online ordering facility.

British Library Cataloguing in Publication Data

A catalogue record for this book is available from the British Library.

ISBN-13: 978 1 84619 227 2

Set and printed by Graphicraft Limited, Hong Kong

Contents

Foreword

Since its initial publication in 2001, *Medical Masterclass* has been regarded as a key learning and teaching resource for physicians around the world. The resource was produced in part to meet the Royal College of Physicians' vision: *'Doctors of the highest quality, serving patients well'*. This vision continues and has led to the compilation of two volumes of self-assessment questions – one of which you now hold in your hands.

The MRCP(UK) is an examination of high international standing and reputation that seeks to advance the learning of, and enhance the training process for, physicians worldwide. On passing the examination physicians are recognised as having attained the required knowledge, skills and manner appropriate for training at a specialist level. However, passing the examination is a challenge. The pass rate at each sitting of the written papers is about 40%. Even the most prominent consultants have had to sit each part of the examination more than once in order to pass. With this challenge in mind, the College and Radcliffe Publishing have produced this compilation of self-assessment questions that were written as part of *Medical Masterclass*, the aim being to help as many doctors as possible in the revision process for the MRCP(UK) examination. I hope you find them to be as beneficial to your studies as thousands of other doctors have; and that you enjoy the challenges they present to your medical knowledge!

Professor Ian Gilmore MD PRCP
President of the Royal College of Physicians
September 2007

Preface

This collection of self-assessment questions and explanatory answers has been drawn from *Medical Masterclass*, which is produced and published by the Education Department of the Royal College of Physicians of London. The questions have been specifically written to help doctors in their first few years of training to test and revise their medical knowledge and skills; and in particular to pass postgraduate examinations, such as the MRCP(UK).

These questions come in the format that is found in both the MRCP(UK) Part 1 or Part 2 examinations. They cover the scientific background to medicine, general clinical skills, acute medicine and the range of medical specialties; all of which candidates will be tested on when they sit their MRCP(UK). The questions collected in this volume will provide a stern test for any such doctor, and how they fare will give them a good indication of where to focus the remainder of their revision if they want to be successful in their upcoming examinations.

I hope that you enjoy using these *Medical Masterclass* self-assessment questions to test your knowledge of medicine, which – whatever is happening politically to primary care, hospitals and medical career structures – remains a wonderful occupation. It is sometimes intellectually and/or emotionally very challenging, and also sometimes extremely rewarding, particularly when reduced to the essential of a doctor trying to provide best care for a patient.

Dr John Firth DM FRCP
Editor-in-Chief
September 2007

List of contributors

Genetics and molecular medicine

Professor Timothy J Vyse MA MRCP(UK) PhD
Honorary Consultant in Rheumatology/Medicine and
Wellcome Trust Senior Fellow
Imperial College London, Faculty of Medicine and
Hammersmith Hospital
London

Biochemistry and metabolism

Dr Fiona M Gribble MA DPhil MRCPath
Wellcome Senior Research Fellow and
Honorary Consultant in Clinical Biochemistry
Cambridge Institute for Medical Research and Department of
Clinical Biochemistry, Addenbrooke's Hospital
Cambridge

Cell biology

Dr Emma H Baker PhD FRCP
Reader and Consultant in Clinical Pharmacology
Division of Basic Medical Sciences
St George's, University of London
London

Dr Kristian M Bowles MB BS PhD MRCP(UK) MRCPath
Consultant Haematologist
Norfolk and Norwich University Hospital NHS Trust
Norwich

Dr Graham G Dark MBBS PhD FRCP
Clinical Senior Lecturer
Northern Centre for Cancer Treatment
Newcastle General Hospital
Newcastle-upon-Tyne

Dr Aroon D Hingorani MA PhD FRCP
Senior Lecturer
Centre for Clinical Pharmacology and Therapeutics
University College London
London

Immunology and immunosuppression

Professor Kevin A Davies BA MBBS MA MD FRCP
Chair of Medicine
Brighton and Sussex Medical School
Brighton

Dr Michael G Robson BA PhD MRCP(UK)
Senior Lecturer and Honorary Consultant Nephrologist
King's College London
London

Anatomy

Dr Samuel Jacob MBBS MS (Anatomy)
Formerly Senior Lecturer
Department of Biomedical Science
University of Sheffield
Sheffield

Physiology

Dr Jane D Collier MB ChB MD FRCP
Consultant Hepatologist
John Radcliffe Hospital
Oxford

Dr Anna Crown MA MB BChir MRCP(UK) PhD
Consultant Endocrinologist and Honorary Senior Lecturer
Bristol and Sussex University Hospitals NHS Trust
Royal Sussex County Hospital
East Sussex

Dr John D Firth DM FRCP
Consultant Physician and Nephrologist
Addenbrooke's Hospital
Cambridge

Dr Peter E Glennon MB ChB Hons MD FRCP
Consultant Cardiologist
University Hospital
Coventry

Dr Mark Gurnell BSc Hons MBBS FRCP PhD
University Lecturer and
Honorary Consultant Physician
University of Cambridge, Department of Medicine
and Addenbrooke's Hospital
Cambridge

Dr Paul R Roberts MB ChB FRCP MD
Consultant Cardiologist
Southampton General Hospital
Southampton

Dr Catherine EG Head MA MRCP(UK) PhD
Consultant Cardiologist
Guy's and St Thomas' NHS Foundation Trust
London

Dr John M Hebden MBBS BSc MD FRCP
Consultant Physician and Gastroenterologist
Northern General Hospital
Sheffield

Dr Michael I Polkey MRCP(UK) PhD
Consultant Physician
Royal Brompton Hospital and
National Heart & Lung Institute
London

Dr Jeremy Shearman DPhil FRCP
Consultant Gastroenterologist
Warwick Hospital
Warwick

Dr Mohammed Z Qureshi MBBS MRCP(UK)
Consultant Physician
Mid Cheshire Hospitals NHS Trust
Crewe, Cheshire

Dr Hamish A Walker BA Hons MBBS MRCP(UK)
Western Infirmary, Glasgow
North Glasgow University Hospitals NHS Trust

Dr Nick S Ward BSc MBBS MRCP(UK)
Consultant Neurologist
National Hospital for Neurology and
Neurosurgery and Institute of Neurology
University College London
London

Clinical pharmacology

Dr Emma H Baker PhD FRCP
Reader and Consultant in Clinical Pharmacology
Division of Basic Medical Sciences
St George's, University of London
London

Dr Stephen F Haydock MA MB BChir PhD FRCP
Consultant Physician and Director of Acute Medical Services
Addenbrooke's Hospital
Cambridge

Dr Aroon D Hingorani MA FRCP PhD
Senior Lecturer
Centre for Clinical Pharmacology and Therapeutics
University College London
London

Dr D John M Reynolds MA BM BCh DPhil FRCP
Consultant Physician and Clinical Pharmacologist
John Radcliffe Hospital
Oxford

Statistics, epidemiology, clinical trials, meta-analyses and evidence-based medicine

Clinical trials and meta-analyses:

Professor John Danesh MB ChB MSc DPhil FRCP
Head, Department of Public Health and Primary Care
University of Cambridge
Cambridge

Evidence-based medicine:

Professor William Rosenberg MA MBBS DPhil FRCP
Professor of Hepatology
Southampton General Hospital
Southampton

Statistics and epidemiology:

Professor Christopher JM Whitty MA MSc FRCP DTM&H
Clinical Research Unit
London School of Hygiene and Tropical Medicine
London

Pain relief and palliative care

Dr G Nicola Rudd MB ChB FRCP
Consultant in Palliative Medicine
Palliative Care Team
Leicester Royal Infirmary
Leicester

Emergency medicine

Dr C Andrew Eynon BSc MBBS FRCP FFAEM
Director of Neurosciences Intensive Care
Wessex Neurological Centre
Southampton General Hospital
Southampton

Professor Paul F Jenkins MA MB BChir FRCP FRCPE
Professor of Acute Medicine
Joondalup Health Campus
Western Australia

Dr Carole M Gavin (nee Libetta) MB ChB MRCP(UK)
FRCS(Ed) FCEM MD
Consultant in Emergency Medicine
Salford Royal Hospitals Foundation Trust
Salford

Infectious diseases

Dr Alec Bonington BSc MB ChB FRCP DTMH MD
Clinical Director and
Consultant in Infectious Diseases
Monsall Unit
Department of Infectious Diseases
North Manchester General Hospital
Manchester

Dr Carolyn Hemsley MRCP(UK) MRCPath BM BCh MA PhD
Consultant in Infectious Diseases and Microbiology
St Thomas' Hospital
London

Dr Michael Jacobs MA PhD FRCP DTMH
Senior Lecturer and
Honorary Consultant in Infectious Diseases
University College London Medical School and
Royal Free Hampstead NHS Trust
London

Dr Paul Klenerman MRCP(UK) DPhil
Wellcome Trust Research Fellow
Nuffield Department of Medicine
University of Oxford
Oxford

Dr William Lynn MBBS MD FRCP
Consultant in Infectious Diseases and Medical Director
Ealing Hospital NHS Trust
London

Dermatology

Dr Karen Harman DM MA MB BChir FRCP
Consultant Dermatologist
University Hospitals of Leicester
Leicester

Dr Graham Ogg BM BCh FRCP DPhil
MRC Senior Clinical Fellow and
Honorary Consultant Dermatologist
Oxford Radcliffe NHS Trust
Oxford

Dr Natalie M Stone BA Hons FRCP
Dermatology Consultant
Royal Gwent NHS Trust
Newport, Gwent

Haematology

Dr Kristian M Bowles MB BS PhD MRCP(UK) MRCPath
Consultant Haematologist
Norfolk and Norwich University Hospital NHS Trust
Norwich

Dr David W Galvani MD MEd FRCP FRCPath
Consultant Haematologist
Haematology Department
Arrowe Park Hospital
Wirral

Dr Bronwen E Shaw MB ChB MRCP(UK)
Haematology Consultant
Royal Marsden Hospital
London

Oncology

Dr Mark Bower FRCP FRCPath PhD
Consultant Medical Oncologist
Department of Oncology
Chelsea & Westminster Hospital
London

Dr Graham G Dark MBBS PhD FRCP
Clinical Senior Lecturer
Northern Centre for Cancer Treatment
Newcastle General Hospital
Newcastle-upon-Tyne

Cardiology

Dr Peter E Glennon MB ChB Hons MD FRCP
Consultant Cardiologist
University Hospital
Coventry

Dr Catherine EG Head MA MRCP(UK) PhD
Consultant Cardiologist
Guy's and St Thomas' NHS Foundation Trust
London

Dr Paul R Roberts MB ChB FRCP MD
Consultant Cardiologist
Southampton General Hospital
Southampton

Dr Hamish A Walker BA Hons MBBS MRCP(UK)
Western Infirmary, Glasgow
North Glasgow University Hospitals NHS Trust

Respiratory medicine

Dr Praveen Bhatia MBBS MRCP(Ireland)
Consultant Physician, Respiratory and Internal Medicine
Tameside General Hospital
Ashton-under-Lyme

Dr Michael I Polkey MRCP(UK) PhD
Consultant Physician
Royal Brompton Hospital and
National Heart & Lung Institute
London

Dr Veronica LC White BSc MSc MBBS FRCP MD
Vascular Physiologist and Clinical Scientist
Barts and the London NHS Trust
London

Gastroenterology and hepatology

Dr Jane D Collier MB ChB MD FRCP
Consultant Hepatologist
John Radcliffe Hospital
Oxford

Dr John M Hebden MBBS BSc MD FRCP
Consultant Physician and Gastroenterologist
Northern General Hospital
Sheffield

Dr Satish Keshav MB BCh DPhil FRCP
Consultant Gastroenterologist
Department of Gastroenterology
John Radcliffe Hospital
Oxford

Dr Jeremy Shearman DPhil FRCP
Consultant Gastroenterologist
Warwick Hospital
Warwick

Neurology

Dr Gillian L Hall BSc BM BCh MRCP(UK) PhD
Consultant Neurologist
Aberdeen Royal Infirmary
Aberdeen

Dr Aroon D Hingorani MA FRCP PhD
Senior Lecturer
Centre for Clinical Pharmacology and Therapeutics
University College London
London

Dr John P Patten BSc FRCP
Latterly Consultant Neurologist
King Edward VII Hospital
Midhurst
West Sussex

Dr Sivakumar Sathasivam MB BCh MRCP(UK) PhD
Consultant Neurologist
The Walton Centre for Neurology & Neurosurgery
Liverpool

Dr Nick S Ward BSc MBBS MRCP(UK)
Consultant Neurologist
National Hospital for Neurology and Neurosurgery and
Institute of Neurology
University College London
London

Ophthalmology

Dr Peggy Frith MD FRCP FRCOphth
Consultant Ophthalmic Physician
Oxford Eye Hospital and University College Hospital,
London

Dr Hamish MA Towler MD FRCPEd FRCSEd FRCOphth
Consultant Ophthalmologist and Lead Clinician
Eye Treatment Centre
Whipps Cross University Hospital
London

Psychiatry

Dr Vincent Kirchner MB ChB FCPsych(SA)
Consultant Psychiatrist
Camden & Islington Mental Health and Social Care NHS Trust
London

Dr Maurice Lipsedge MPhil FRCP FRCPsych FFOM(Hon)
Emeritus Consultant Psychiatrist
The South London and Maudsley NHS Trust
Visiting Senior Lecturer
Department of Psychological Medicine, Guy's, King's and
St Thomas' School of Medicine

Endocrinology

Dr Anna Crown MA MB BChir MRCP(UK) PhD
Consultant Endocrinologist and
Honorary Senior Lecturer
Bristol and Sussex University Hospitals NHS Trust
Royal Sussex County Hospital
East Sussex

Dr Paul D Flynn MA MB BChir MRCP(UK) MRCPI PhD
Consultant Physician in Acute & Metabolic Medicine
Addenbrooke's Hospital
Cambridge

Dr M Gurnell BSc Hons MBBS FRCP PhD
University Lecturer and Honorary Consultant Physician
University of Cambridge, Department of Medicine and
Addenbrooke's Hospital
Cambridge

Dr Mohammed Z Qureshi MBBS MRCP(UK)
Consultant Physician
Mid Cheshire Hospitals NHS Trust
Crewe, Cheshire

Nephrology

Dr Nick C Fluck MBBS BSc FRCP DPhil
Consultant Nephrologist and Unit Clinical Director
Medical Renal Unit
Aberdeen Royal Infirmary
Aberdeen

Dr Philip A Kalra MA MB BChir FRCP MD
Consultant Nephrologist and
Honorary Senior Lecturer
Hope Hospital, Salford and
University of Manchester

Professor Patrick H Maxwell FRCP MA MBBS DPhil FMedSci
Chair of Nephrology
Imperial College London
London

Dr Chris A O'Callaghan BA BM BCh MA MRCP(UK) DPhil
Reader and Consultant Nephrologist
Nuffield Department of Medicine and Oxford Kidney Unit
University of Oxford and Churchill Hospital Oxford
Oxford

Rheumatology and clinical immunology

Dr Khalid Binymin MB ChB FRCP MSc
Consultant Physician and Rheumatologist
Southport and Ormskirk NHS Trust
Southport

Dr Hilary J Longhurst MA FRCP PhD FRCPath
Consultant Immunologist and Lead Clinician
Immunopathology and Clinical Immunology
St Bartholomew's Hospital and the London NHS Trust
London

Dr Siraj A Misbah MBBS MSc FRCP FRCPath
Consultant Clinical Immunologist and
Honorary Senior Clinical Lecturer in Immunology
Oxford Radcliffe Hospitals NHS Trust and
University of Oxford
Churchill and John Radcliffe Hospitals
Oxford

Dr Neil Snowden MB BChir FRCP FRCPath
Consultant Rheumatologist and Clinical Immunologist
North Manchester General Hospital
Manchester

Questions

Genetics and molecular medicine

Timothy J Vyse

Genetics and Molecular Medicine

Answers are on pp. 125–126.

Question 1
In the field of molecular biology, the term imprinting means:
A the tendency of some diseases to get more severe as they pass from generation to generation
B that two genes are associated and therefore inherited together
C the differential expression of alleles contingent on their parental origin
D that one allele of a gene is not expressed
E that a gene is inherited from the mitochondrial genome

Question 2
In the field of molecular biology, the term recombination means the:
A coming together of chromosomes at meiosis
B separation of chromosomes at mitosis
C combination of alleles from both parents at fertilisation
D production of genetic combinations not found in either of the parents
E tendency of some genetic disorders to run true in families

Question 3
In the field of molecular biology, if a putative gene for a disease trait and a known genetic locus are linked with a LOD score of 3.0, this means the probability that the putative gene is linked to the known genetic locus is:
A 3 : 1
B 300 : 1
C 1,000 : 1
D 3,000 : 1
E 3,000,000 : 1

Question 4
In the field of molecular biology, a codon is a:
A 3-base pair unit of DNA that codes for an amino acid
B 3-base pair unit of RNA that codes for an amino acid
C 4-base pair unit of DNA that codes for an amino acid
D 4-base pair unit of RNA that codes for an amino acid
E 4-base pair unit of DNA that codes for a 4-base pair unit of RNA

Question 5
In the field of molecular biology, the term 'TATA box' refers to:
A a DNA sequence often found in the promoter element (start) of a gene
B a DNA sequence often found in the transcriptional stop site (end) of a gene
C an RNA sequence often found at the 5 prime end (start) of an RNA message
D an RNA sequence often found at the 3 prime end (finish) of an RNA message
E a DNA sequence that leads to splicing of an RNA transcript.

Question 6
A Mendelian X-linked dominant condition would be transmitted to:
A all of the sons of an affected woman
B all children of an affected man
C none of the sons of an affected woman
D all of the sons of an affected man
E half of the daughters of an affected woman

Question 7
Regarding the polymerase chain reaction (PCR), which one of the following statements is true?
A PCR can be used directly on any form of nucleic acid to obtain multiple copies thereof
B PCR is not of diagnostic use, as the enzyme employed in the reaction is very prone to error
C PCR utilises DNA polymerases that are stable at low temperature but denature at high temperature
D PCR is a useful means of characterising genetic markers
E PCR results in a linear amplification of starting material, so that after 30 cycles of PCR the amount of material generated would be 30 times the amount of starting material

Question 8
Considering the use of animal models in the investigation of human genetic disease, which one of the following statements is correct?

5

A primates are widely used to model human genetic disease

B mice are a good model for a range of human central nervous system diseases

C a transgenic mouse is one in which a critical region of a gene has been removed so that the gene product exerts no or little function

D making a 'knock-out' mouse involves deleting or altering a gene sequence in an unfertilised egg

E large regions of human and rodent genomes encode structurally and functionally related genes

Question 9

Consider the scenario of two separate genetic loci A and B, where each locus carries two possible alleles. If these two loci A and B are in linkage disequilibrium, which one of the following statements is true?

A the four alleles at A and B are inherited independently provided that the population is of sufficient size

B the inheritance of an allele at A will almost certainly exclude the inheritance of one of the alleles at B

C it is most likely that the least common alleles will be in linkage disequilibrium

D the loci A and B are likely to be linked

E patterns of linkage disequilibrium in a northern European population will, in the vast majority of cases, be reproduced in a northern Indo-Asian population

Question 10

Considering the structure of nucleic acids, which one of the following statements is true?

A in DNA the two purine bases pair with one another, and the two pyrimidine bases pair with one another

B in RNA, the 2' and 3' carbon atoms of ribose are hydroxylated

C DNA is inherently more unstable than RNA

D when RNA is copied (transcribed) from DNA, a guanine copies cytosine, and a thymine copies adenine

E in non-sex chromosomes (autosomes) both maternal and paternal alleles always contribute to the gene product

Biochemistry and metabolism

Fiona M Gribble

Biochemistry and Metabolism

Answers are on pp. 126–128.

Question 11
Amino acids are linked together in proteins by peptide bonds, which are:
A bonds between the carboxylic acid group of one amino acid and the amino group of the next
B bonds between the amino group of one amino acid and the amino group of the next
C bonds between the carboxylic acid group of one amino acid and the carboxylic acid group of the next
D bonds between alternating purine and pyrimidine amino acids
E hydrogen bonds between side chains of amino acids

Question 12
Which one of the following is the best description of glycogen? Chains of glucose residues linked by:
A alpha-1,4 glycosidic bonds
B alpha-1,4 glycosidic bonds with branches formed by alpha-1,6 glycosidic linkages
C alpha-1,6 glycosidic bonds
D alpha-1,6 glycosidic bonds with branches formed by alpha-1,4 glycosidic linkages
E alternating alpha-1,4 and alpha-1,6 glycosidic bonds

Question 13
Which one of the following statements best describes the synthesis of fatty acids? Fatty acids are built up from:
A acetyl CoA units in the mitochondrion
B cholesterol units in the mitochondrion
C acetyl CoA units in the cytosol
D cholesterol units in the cytosol
E alternating acetyl CoA and cholesterol units in the mitochondrial outer membrane

Question 14
Glycosaminoglycans form a major part of the ground substance of connective tissue. They are made of chains of:
A glucose
B glucosamine
C glucuronic acid
D disaccharides
E amino acids

Question 15
Which one of the following is a direct product of the pentose phosphate pathway?
A NADH
B NADPH
C Glucose-6-phosphate
D ATP
E Acetyl CoA

Question 16
Which one of the following amino acids has a positively charged side chain at physiological pH?
A arginine
B glutamine
C methionine
D glutamate
E threonine

Question 17
Which of the following is an essential amino acid?
A alanine
B cysteine
C leucine
D glutamine
E tyrosine

Question 18
Which one of the following statements about alpha-helices in proteins is correct?
A they can only be composed of amino acids without bulky side chains
B the side chains project outwards from the axis of the helix
C a high proportion of charged residues often indicates the position of a transmembrane domain
D the structure of collagen is an example of an alpha-helix
E proline residues are a common finding within alpha-helices

Question 19

Which one of the following statements about protein synthesis is correct?

A translation always begins with a methionine residue

B ricin is an inhibitor of eukaryotic transcription

C ribosome binding to the poly-A tail of mRNA is involved in the initiation of translation

D translation proceeds along the mRNA in the 3′ to 5′ direction

E new amino acids are added to the N-terminus of the growing peptide chain

Question 20

Which one of the following CANNOT be converted to glucose by gluconeogenesis?

A glycerol

B alanine

C lactate

D acetyl CoA produced by beta-oxidation of fatty acids

E glutamine

Cell biology

**Emma H Baker, Kristian M Bowles,
Graham G Dark and Aroon D Hingorani**

Cell Biology

Answers are on pp. 128–130.

Question 21
Regarding the action of steroids, which one of the following statements is true?
A steroids act by binding to membrane-bound receptors
B steroids act by modifying gene transcription
C steroid action involves conversion of GTP to cyclic GMP
D steroid action involves binding with G-protein-coupled receptors
E steroid action is mediated by cAMP

Question 22
In neurones, membrane stabilisation is achieved by stimulation of GABA receptors which opens associated Cl⁻ channels. Action potentials are initiated when changes in membrane potential activate opening of voltage-gated Na⁺ channels. Drugs that stimulate GABA receptors have anti-epileptic actions through which one of the following mechanisms?
A they reduce Na⁺ influx into the neurone
B they increase Na⁺ influx into the neurone
C they reduce Cl⁻ influx into the neurone
D they depolarise the neuronal membrane
E they reduce the threshold for action potentials

Question 23
Regarding apoptosis, which one of the following statements is true?
A it occurs whenever a cell dies
B it is reversible in some circumstances
C a key feature in the mechanism is a fall in intracellular calcium concentration
D p53 is an important initiator
E DNA is cleaved into very small fragments (< 10 base pairs)

Question 24
Regarding the cell cycle, which one of the following statements is true?
A most cells in adult tissues are in the S phase, where DNA synthesis occurs
B meiosis completes the cell cycle
C errors during DNA replication are repaired during G0
D there are six phases to the cell cycle
E phosphorylation of the retinoblastome gene product (Rb) promotes progression through G1

Question 25
Regarding the Na/K-ATPase transporter, which one of the following statements is true?
A it is composed of dimers of alpha subunits
B it is present in the membranes of all living cells in the body, excepting red blood cells
C it is largely responsible for maintaining the cell's resting membrane potential
D it transports two sodium ions out of the cell for every two potassium ions pumped into the cell
E it is stimulated by digoxin

Question 26
Which one of the following statements concerning tumour necrosis factor alpha (TNFα) is FALSE?
A the major cellular sources of TNFα are lymphocytes and platelets
B the gene encoding TNFα is located in the MHC region
C TNFα polymorphisms are associated with prognosis in septic shock
D TNFα polymorphisms are associated with susceptibility to cerebral malaria
E biological agents that inhibit TNF are sometimes used in patients with rheumatoid arthritis

Question 27
Nitric oxide exerts its biological effect by:
A interacting with a cell surface G-protein-coupled receptor
B interacting with a cell surface receptor with integral enzymatic function
C activating cytosolic guanylate cyclase
D activating a receptor tyrosine kinase
E binding to a cytosolic receptor that modifies gene transcription

Question 28
Protein kinase C is activated by:
A cAMP
B cCMP
C cGMP
D diacylglycerol
E acetyl choline

Question 29
Thiazide diuretics exert their main action by interacting with which one of the following:
A Na/K ATPase
B Na channel
C Na/H antiporter
D NaK2Cl co-transporter
E NaCl co-transporter

Question 30
The rapid depolarisation of the action potential is caused by:
A Entry of sodium through voltage-gated sodium channels
B Exit of sodium through voltage-gated sodium channels
C Entry of calcium through voltage-gated calcium channels
D Entry of potassium through voltage-gated potassium channels
E Exit of potassium through voltage-gated potassium channels

Immunology and immunosuppression

Kevin A Davies and Michael G Robson

Immunology and Immunosuppression

Answers are on pp. 130–131.

Question 31
Which one of the following statements about the T cell receptor is true?
A unlike B cell receptors (antibody), the T cell receptor gene does not get rearranged during development
B it is comprised of three chains
C on the cell surface it is not associated with CD3
D one T cell may express more than one specificity of T cell receptor
E on the cell surface it may be associated with CD4 or CD8

Question 32
Which one of the following statements does NOT correctly link an immunosuppressive drug with its mechanism of action?
A cyclosporin (ciclosporin) and calineurin inhibition
B tacrolimus and calcineurin inhibition
C tacrolimus and FKBP12
D rapamycin (sirolimus) and FKBP12
E azathioprine and inosine monophosphate dehydrogenase inhibition

Question 33
Which one of the following types of cell does NOT develop in the bone marrow?
A neutrophils
B monocytes
C B cells
D T cells
E platelets

Question 34
Which one of the following is NOT a component of the cytolytic granules found in cytotoxic T cells and NK cells?
A granulysins
B perforins
C granzyme A
D granzyme B
E membrane attack complex

Question 35
Which one of the following statements regarding defects in inflammatory and immune responses is true?
A X-linked agammaglobulinaemia usually presents in early adulthood
B selective IgA deficiency is treated with intravenous gammaglobulin (IVIG)
C chronic granulomatous disease is due to impaired neutrophil phagocytosis
D common variable immunodeficiency (CVID) is associated with autoimmune disease
E defects in the classical pathway of complement predispose to Neisserial infections

Question 36
T-helper cells have:
A CD4 on their surface and recognise peptides presented on MHC class I molecules
B CD8 on their surface and recognise peptides presented on MHC class I molecules
C CD8 on their surface and recognise peptides presented on MHC class II molecules
D CD4 on their surface and recognise peptides presented on MHC class II molecules
E CD8 on their surface and recognise peptides presented on the CD4 molecule

Question 37
T cells are divided into Th1 and Th2 depending on the pattern of effector cytokines they produce. Which of the following is a Th1 cytokine?
A interleukin 13
B interferon gamma
C interleukin 4
D interleukin 10
E interleukin 6

Question 38
The cells of the immune system may be divided into those that are important in innate immunity and those involved in adaptive immunity. Which one of the following is not involved in innate immunity?

A macrophage
B neutrophil
C NK cell
D B cell
E eosinophil

Question 39
Which one of the following is a membrane bound complement inhibitor?
A factor H
B C4 binding protein
C C1 inhibitor
D CD 59
E factor I

Question 40
Which one of the following statements regarding antigen processing is correct?
A TAP molecules are involved in processing molecules presented by MHC class I
B the invariant chain is a well-conserved molecule that is structurally similar to major histocompatibility complex (MHC) class II
C proteosomes are involved in processing molecules presented by MHC class II
D class II molecules typically present peptides from antigen that has been newly synthesized
E MHC class III molecules are functionally and structurally related to MHC class I and II

Anatomy

Samuel Jacob

Anatomy

Answers are on pp. 131–132.

Question 41
The chorda tympani of the facial nerve (cranial nerve VII) carries:
A sympathetic fibres to the submandibular and sublingual glands and taste fibres from the anterior two-thirds of the tongue
B parasympathetic fibres to the submandibular and sublingual glands and the nerve to stapedius
C parasympathetic fibres to the submandibular and sublingual glands and taste fibres from the anterior two-thirds of the tongue
D sympathetic fibres to the submandibular and sublingual glands and taste fibres from the whole of the tongue
E sympathetic fibres to the submandibular and sublingual glands and the nerve to stapedius

Question 42
The vestibulocochlear nerve (cranial nerve VIII) enters the internal acoustic meatus and passes to the cochlear nucleus in the brain stem. Which one of the following pathways correctly describes the pathway by which auditory information then passes to the brain?
A inferior colliculus – lateral lemniscus – lateral geniculate body
B inferior colliculus – lateral lemniscus – medial geniculate body
C superior colliculus – medial lemniscus – medial geniculate body
D superior colliculus – medial lemniscus – lateral geniculate body
E superior colliculus – lateral lemniscus – medial geniculate body

Question 43
Regarding the portal vein, which one of the following statements is true?
A about 25% of the total blood supply of the liver reaches it via the portal vein
B the capillaries of the portal vein in the liver are known as the sinusoids
C blood leaves the liver through branches of the portal vein that join the inferior vena cava
D normal portal pressure is about 12 mmHg
E thrombosis of the portal vein causes Budd–Chiari syndrome

Question 44
With regard to the common bile duct, which of the following statement is NOT true?
A it is formed by the union of common hepatic duct and the cystic duct
B the ampulla of Vater is formed by its union with the pancreatic duct
C the sphincter of Oddi surrounds the ampulla
D the ampulla opens on the papilla of Vater
E the ampulla opens into the duodenum about 5 cms distal to the pylorus

Question 45
Which one of the following statements regarding the lung and pleura is NOT true?
A the lung apex extends about 3 cm above the medial part of the clavicle
B the horizontal fissure separates the right middle lobe from the right lower lobe
C the horizontal fissure may be visible on a plain radiograph of the chest
D the lower margin of the pleura is about two ribs below the lower margin of the lung
E the lower parts of the lung and pleura overlap the right surface of the liver

Question 46
Regarding the apex beat, which one of the following statements is true?
A the apex beat is always palpable
B it is normally felt in the midaxillary line when lying in the left lateral position
C a displaced apex is always a sign of left ventricular enlargement
D a heaving apex beat indicates left ventricular pressure overload
E obese patients will have a tapping apex beat

Question 47

Regarding the parathyroid glands, which of the following statements is true?

A there are usually two parathyroid glands, one on either side of the thyroid gland

B they develop from the third and fourth branchial pouches

C they lie on either side of the thyroid gland

D the parathyroid arteries are branches of the external carotid

E about 3–4% of patients undergoing thyroidectomy develop hypocalcaemia

Question 48

With regard to the anatomy of the bronchial tree, which one of the following statements is true?

A there are about 25 generations of bronchi and bronchioles between the trachea and the alveoli

B the left main bronchus is more vertical than the right one

C the left main bronchus divides into three lobar bronchi, whereas the right only into two

D the bronchi and bronchioles have walls consisting of cartilage and smooth muscles

E walls of the terminal bronchioles have submucosal glands

Question 49

Concerning the functional anatomy of the eye, which one of the following statements is true?

A paralysis of the orbicularis oculi causes ptosis

B the refractory index of the lens is lower than that of vitreous humour

C the choroid plexus produces aqueous humour

D aqueous humour is secreted by the Canal of Schlemm

E tension of the suspensory ligament flattens the lens

Question 50

Regarding the testis, which one of the following statements is true?

A the testis develops in the pelvis and descends to the scrotum

B the right testis is usually at a lower level than the left

C tumours of the testis often spread by lymphatics to the external iliac nodes

D the spermatic cord contains the ductus deferens

E the epididymis lies on the anterior aspect of the testis

Physiology

Jane D Collier, Anna Crown,
John D Firth *(Editor)*, Peter E Glennon,
Mark Gurnell, Paul R Roberts,
Catherine EG Head, John M Hebden,
Michael I Polkey, Jeremy Shearman,
Mohammed Z Qureshi, Hamish A Walker
and Nick Ward

Physiology

Answers are on pp. 132–135.

Question 51

Regarding the action potential of ventricular cardiac myocytes, which one of the following statements is true?

A calcium entry contributes to the plateau phase of the cardiac action potential

B the resting intracellular membrane potential is around +80 mV with respect to the extracellular potential

C it is principally sodium ions that determine the resting membrane potential

D initial depolarization occurs when potassium conductance increases

E chloride exit contributes to the early part of repolarization

Question 52

With regard to pulmonary physiology, which one of the following statements is FALSE?

A following a normal expiration the lungs still contain 3 L of air

B the dead space in an adult is approximately 500 mL

C the diaphragm is supplied from the C3, C4 and C5 nerve roots

D the functional residual capacity is greater than the residual volume

E the residual volume is approximately 1.5 L in an adult

Question 53

Which one of the following statements about aldosterone is NOT true?

A production of aldosterone is directly stimulated by hyperkalaemia

B the main site of action of aldosterone is the collecting duct

C aldosterone binds to a receptor on the cell surface

D aldosterone stimulates increased numbers and activity of the apical ENaC channel

E aldosterone stimulates increased activity of the potassium channel ROMK

Question 54

In the treatment of hyperkalaemia:

A intravenous calcium rapidly lowers the serum potassium concentration

B if the ECG shows severe changes (sine wave pattern), give glucose and insulin as first line treatment

C nebulised salbutamol (10 mg) reduces serum potassium concentration by 1–2 mmol/l over 20–30 min

D calcium resonium can be given intravenously, orally or rectally

E peritoneal dialysis is often used as emergency treatment on renal units

Question 55

The clearance of a substance can be used to calculate glomerular filtration rate if it is:

A not filtered at the glomerulus

B metabolised completely by the kidney

C not reabsorbed or secreted by the renal tubules

D is reabsorbed but not secreted by the renal tubules

E is secreted but not reabsorbed by the renal tubules

Question 56

Regarding the mechanism of sodium handling in the kidney:

A the Na/K/2Cl co-transporter is found in the collecting duct

B most sodium is reabsorbed in the loop of Henle

C aldosterone binds to a receptor on the surface of cells in the collecting duct

D thiazide diuretics interact with a Na/Cl co-transporter in the proximal convoluted tubule

E the Na/K-ATPase is located along the basolateral border of tubular cells

Question 57

Which one of the following statements about cardiac troponins is correct?

A troponins are bound to both thick and thin filaments of the myofibril

B troponins are bound to the thick filaments of the myofibril

C troponin I inhibits contraction

D troponin C causes contraction

E troponin T terminates contraction

Question 58

The R wave of the ECG occurs

A just before mitral valve closure

B just before mitral valve opening

C just before aortic valve closure

D at the mid-point of systole

E at the mid-point of diastole

Question 59

Blood pressure (BP), cardiac output (CO) and total peripheral resistance (TPR) are related according to the formula:

A $BP = CO / TPR$

B $BP = CO \times TPR$

C $BP = TPR / CO$

D $TPR = BP \times CO$

E $TPR = BP / CO$

Question 60

The relationship between resistance to flow through a blood vessell and its radius (r) is proportional to:

A $1/r$

B $1/r^2$

C $1/r^3$

D $1/r^4$

E $1/r^5$

Question 61

In the regulation of vascular tone, nitric oxide is produced from

A alanine

B arginine

C asparagine

D methionine

E phenylalanine

Question 62

Which one of the following is NOT an effect of cholecystokinin:

A inhibition of gastric emptying

B contraction of gall bladder

C stimulation of pancreatic secretion of proteases

D stimulation of pancreatic secretion of lipases

E stimulation of pancreatic secretion of bicarbonate

Question 63

Regarding a patient with jaundice, which one of the following statements is true:

A there can be no urobilinogen in the urine if jaundice is caused by biliary obstruction

B in Gilbert's syndrome there is conjugated hyperbilirubinaemia

C if the gall bladder is palpable, then the jaundice is probably due to obstruction caused by gall stone

D in Dubin-Johnson syndrome there is unconjugated hyperbilirubinaemia

E tenderness to palpation of the right upper quadrant indicates that jaundice is probably due to obstruction caused by gall stone

Question 64

The sodium-potassium (Na/K) ATPase pump transports

A one sodium ion out of the cell for every one potassium ion transported in

B two sodium ions out of the cell for every one potassium ion transported in

C one sodium ion out of the cell for every two potassium ions transported in

D two sodium ions out of the cell for every three potassium ions transported in

E three sodium ions out of the cell for every two potassium ions transported in

Question 65

Interaction of a neurotransmitter with its appropriate receptor causes a local synaptic potential, which can be depolarising or hyperpolarising, depending on whether the postsynaptic membrane potential becomes more or less negative. An inhibitory postsynaptic potential results in increased permeability to only:

A sodium ions

B potassium ions

C chloride ions

D potassium and chloride ions

E sodium and chloride ions

Question 66

The neurotransmitter active at the neuromuscular junction is:

A adrenalin (epinephrine)

B noradrenalin (norepinephrine)

C gamma-amino butyric acid (GABA)

D acetylcholine

E dopamine

Question 67
The anabolic actions of growth hormone are mediated through insulin-like growth factor 1 (IGF1). IGF1 is produced in:
A small intestine
B large intestine
C all tissues except the brain
D liver
E fat

Question 68
Mineralocorticoids are produced by which part of the adrenal gland:
A zona glomerulosa
B zona fasciculata
C zona reticularis
D medulla
E zona glomerulosa, fasciculata and reticularis

Question 69
Which one of the following is NOT a recognised stimulus for ADH secretion
A increase in blood osmolality
B intravascular volume depletion
C nausea
D pain
E constipation

Question 70
When the kidneys excrete an acid load, about 75% is excreted in the form of ammonium. The immediate source of ammonium ions for excretion is:
A alanine
B arginine
C glutamine
D glycine
E serine

Clinical pharmacology

Emma H Baker, Stephen F Haydock,
Aroon D Hingorani and
D John M Reynolds *(Editor)*

Clinical Pharmacology

Answers are on pp. 135–137.

Question 71

A 45-year-old man is taking long-term theophylline for asthma. One evening, he is admitted to the Accident and Emergency department with convulsions. You suspect theophylline toxicity. Which one of the following statements is true?

A his convulsions should not be treated until a theophylline level is available

B theophylline toxicity may have been precipitated by the concomitant prescription of phenytoin

C theophylline toxicity may have been precipitated by the concomitant prescription of erythromycin

D theophylline toxicity only occurs in the elderly

E theophylline is an example of a drug with a wide therapeutic range (therapeutic index)

Question 72

A 60-year-old woman is admitted feeling generally unwell. Her serum potassium is found to be elevated at 7.0 mmol/l. Which of the following drugs is the LEAST likely to have contributed to her hyperkalaemia?

A lisinopril

B bendrofluazide

C losartan

D spironolactone

E slow-release potassium chloride

Question 73

A 40-year-old woman has developed haemolytic anaemia secondary to drug therapy. Which of the following drugs is NOT a well-recognised cause of haemolytic anaemia?

A phenoxymethylpenicillin

B mefenamic acid

C methyldopa

D ranitidine

E rifampicin

Question 74

A 52-year-old lady who is on some regular medication presents with a sore throat and fever. You check a full blood count and find that the patient has developed neutropenia. Which of the following drugs is most likely to have caused this side effect?

A captopril

B carbimazole

C carvedilol

D ciprofloxacin

E clomipramine

Question 75

A 65-year-old gentleman attending the cardiology clinic complains of swelling and tenderness of his breasts. You diagnose probable gynaecomastia. Which of the following drugs is most likely to be the cause?

A Simvastatin

B Amiodarone

C Digoxin

D Aspirin

E Ramipril

Question 76

A patient presents with acute dystonia and oculogyric crisis after being treated with metoclopramide. Which statement is true with regards to this adverse drug reaction?

A it occurs only after long-term use of metoclopramide

B it is most common in middle-aged men

C it can persist for several days after withdrawal

D it does not occur with prochlorperazine

E it is best treated with procyclidine

Question 77

A patient has developed abnormal thyroid function tests after being started on amiodarone two months ago. Which one of the following features, in conjunction with clinical symptoms and signs, is helpful in diagnosing overt hypothyroidism?

A increase in thyroid-stimulating hormone (TSH) up to 20 mU/L

B decrease in T3

C elevated free T4 and T3

D T4 at upper end of or just above normal range

E low free T4, and low T3

Question 78

A 17-year-old boy fails to breathe spontaneously after an operation. Talking to his family, his sister has previously had similar problems. Which of the following drugs could have caused this problem?

A thiopentone

B atracurium

C suxamethonium

D cisatracurium

E halothane

Question 79

A 58-year-old man with elevated cholesterol has failed to reach a desired cholesterol level on statin treatment. You decide to commence him on ezetimibe. Which of the following is true concerning ezetimibe?

A prescription with statin treatment is contraindicated

B decreased absorption of fat soluble vitamins is an unwanted effect

C its main action is to prevent cholesterol synthesis by the liver

D it causes an elevation in plasma triglyceride concentrations

E it causes a reduction in low-density lipoprotein (LDL)-cholesterol of approximately 20%

Question 80

A 73-year-old man with dementia attends clinic with his wife. She has heard about memantine and wonders if it would be suitable for her husband. Which one of the following is true of memantine?

A it has no interaction with amantadine

B it is licensed for patients with all types of dementia

C it inhibits renal excretion of ranitidine

D it enhances the effects of barbiturates

E it is an acteylcholinesterase inhibitor

Question 81

A 24-year-old Type I diabetic is currently on a basal-bolus regime, comprising twice daily basal isophane insulin complemented by short-acting insulin at meal times. He has recently heard about insulin glargine and wonders if it would be suitable for him. Which statement concerning insulin glargine is true?

A it is formulated by adding zinc suspension to insulin

B it is rapid-acting and should be injected just before meals

C it is particularly useful for patients troubled by hypo-glycaemic episodes

D it needs to be mixed thoroughly before injecting

E it has little effect on fasting blood glucose

Question 82

A 72-year-old white woman has uncomplicated essential hypertension. Her blood pressure is 162/102 mmHg despite optimization of non-pharmacological therapy. Which one of the following would you choose as the first-line treatment for her?

A atenolol 50 od

B bendrofluazide 2.5 mg od

C bendrofluazide 5 mg od

D enalapril 5 mg od

E ramipril 2.5 mg od

Question 83

A 48-year-old Afro-Caribbean man has uncomplicated essential hypertension with blood pressure 154/102 mmHg despite optimization of non-pharmacological therapy. Which one of the following would you use as the first-line treatment in this patient?

A atenolol 50 mg od

B nifedipine 10 mg tds

C amlodipine 5 mg od

D ramipril 2.5 mg od

E enalapril 5 mg bd

Question 84

A middle-aged man is brought by ambulance to the Medical Admissions Unit. He was fitting when picked up and is still having a grand mal convulsion. The most appropriate treatment is:

A lorazepam 2 mg intravenously

B fosphenytoin 15 mg/kg body weight phenytoin equivalent, intravenously at a rate of 100–150 mg phenytoin equivalent/min

C phenytoin 15 mg/kg body weight, intravenously at a rate of 50 mg/min

D diazepam 10 mg intravenously

E phenobarbitone 10 mg/kg body weight, intravenously at a rate of 100 mg/min

Question 85

In a healthy volunteer study, the diuretic response to intravenous doses of loop diuretics A, B and C were compared. A 1 mg dose of diuretic A produced a similar diuresis to 40 mg of diuretic B and 50 mcg of diuretic C. It was found that maximal doses of A produced a similar diuresis to maximal doses of B, but the response obtained with maximal doses of C was considerably lower than that of A or B. Which of the following statements is correct in relation to the action of A, B and C:

A drugs A and B are of similar potency

B drug C is more potent than drug A but of lower efficacy

C drug C is of lower potency than drugs A and B but of greater efficacy

D drug A is of greater efficacy than drugs B and C

E no conclusion can be drawn regarding the relative efficacy and potency of the three drugs

Statistics, epidemiology, clinical trials, meta-analyses and evidence-based medicine

John Danesh, William Rosenberg and
Christopher JM Whitty

Statistics, Epidemiology, Clinical Trials, Meta-analyses and Evidence-based Medicine

Answers are on pp. 137–141.

Question 86

In the field of statistics, which of the following statements regarding a forest plot is true?

A the area of the squares is proportional to the number of events in each study

B the lengths of the horizontal lines emerging from the squares represent standard deviations

C the lengths of the horizontal lines emerging from the squares represent two standard deviations

D the area of the squares is proportional to the magnitude of the treatment effect in each study

E it is a method of combining data when individual studies are of insufficient power to show an effect

Question 87

In the field of statistics, a factorial trial means that:

A two or more treatments are tested sequentially

B two or more treatments are tested simultaneously

C the patients in the trial are stratified into two or more groups

D each patient receives one active drug and one placebo treatment

E the trial takes more than one factor into account

Question 88

The following is a description of a test. "The new test has a sensitivity of 99% and a specificity of 83%. In those under 65 years old it has a positive predictive value of 48%". A test with these characteristics would NOT be appropriate in which one of the following situations?

A rapid screening for HIV in a same-day-result STI clinic

B screening anonymously donated blood for HIV before transfusion

C as a preliminary part of a medical assessment looking for heart disease in potential army recruits

D a screening test for head lice in children

E as an indication for sigmoidoscopy and barium enema for lower gastrointestinal malignancy in patients with chronic diarrhoea

Question 89

Concerning cohort studies, which one of the following statements is true?

A they can only be used to compare two groups with one another

B they are particularly useful with rare outcomes

C cohort studies are retrospective

D they are better than other study types for measuring the incidence of a disease in a population

E they are better than other study designs for measuring prevalence of a disease in a population

Question 90

Concerning the statistical power of studies, which one of the following statements is FALSE?

A a power calculation must always be performed before conducting randomized clinical trials

B a type II error occurs if it is claimed two treatments are the same when the study is not large enough to detect equivalence

C a type I error is where the null hypothesis is falsely rejected

D the smaller the difference you want to detect, the larger a study must be

E international journals do not publish studies that are underpowered

Question 91

Regarding crossover trial design, which one of the following statements is true?

A it can be used to compare treatments for an acute infection

B it cannot be double-blinded

C it cannot be randomised

D it is a good method for comparing analgesics in arthritis

E tends to need more patients than are required with other trial designs to get adequate statistical power

Question 92
Regarding case-control studies, which one of the following statements is FALSE?
A they are good for investigating rare diseases
B they are good for identifying rare causes of disease
C they may be uninterpretable if controls are selected poorly
D they can examine multiple risk-factors for a single disease
E they compare exposures of interest in cases and controls

Question 93
For continuous data, which one of the following statements is true?
A a positive s test (skew test) result means that the data is not normally distributed
B it is always wrong to use the mean to describe skewed data
C chi-squared is the best test for comparing skewed continuous data
D the Wilcoxon rank-sum test is best used with normally distributed data
E the interquartile range is two standard deviations wide

Question 94
The practice of evidence-based medicine (EBM) begins with the formulation of an answerable question. Which one of the following elements is NOT required for a question to be answerable?
A a particular patient or problem
B an intervention
C a comparison
D an outcome measure
E at least one relevant randomised controlled trial

Question 95
The statistical reviewer of a paper states that they are concerned that the findings are biased. In statistical terms, 'bias' means:
A there is a flaw in study design that leads to a built-in likelihood that the wrong result may be obtained
B there is a flaw in statistical analysis leading to a likelihood that the wrong result may be obtained
C there is reason to believe that the authors wanted to obtain the result that the study showed
D both study design and statistical analysis are flawed, leading to a likelihood that the wrong result may be obtained

E the study is not of sufficient statistical power to exclude the missing of a significant effect

Question 96
A researcher is trying to design a study to find out the cause (or causes) of a rare disease, about which very little is known. What study design is most likely to be appropriate?
A geographical
B cross-sectional
C cohort
D intervention
E case control

Question 97
A 95% confidence interval means:
A 95% of the data fall within the confidence interval
B there is a 95% chance that two groups are different
C that $p = 0.05$
D there is a 95% chance that the true value falls within the confidence interval
E there is a 95% chance that the finding is clinically significant

Question 98
Regarding the description and comparison of two groups of data, which one of the following statements is true?
A categorical data should be described as percentages and compared using a Student's t-test
B normally distributed continuous data should be described as median and range and compared using a chi-squared test
C skewed continuous data should be described as median and range and compared using a Wilcoxon rank-sum test
D normally distributed continuous data should be described as mean and standard deviation and compared using a chi-squared test
E skewed continuous data should be described as mean and standard deviation and compared using a Student's t-test

Question 99
A manuscript is submitted to a medical journal regarding a randomised trial in which a new treatment for Clostridium difficile diarrhoea is compared with an established treatment. A reviewer states that they are concerned that there might be type 2 statistical error. What does this mean? That the:

A method of statistical analysis used is inappropriate

B study has shown a difference between the treatments that is statistically significant but which is unlikely to be clinically significant

C study claims to find a difference that does not really exist, i.e. the result is a statistical fluke

D data is skewed (not normally distributed) and analysis should have used non-parametric rather than parametric statistical techniques

E study claims that there is no difference between the treatments, when in reality the trial was just too small to detect a difference

Question 100

A placebo-controlled study randomised 10 000 patients undergoing surgery for hip fracture to 160 mg aspirin/day, started preoperatively and continued for 35 days. About 1.5% of the patients allocated aspirin had DVT or pulmonary embolism (PE), compared with about 2.5% allocated placebo. Which one of the following statements about this trial is true?

A aspirin produced a 1.5% absolute risk reduction in DVT/PE

B aspirin produced a 40% absolute risk reduction in DVT/PE

C aspirin produced a 1% proportional risk reduction in DVT/PE

D aspirin produced a 40% proportional risk reduction in DVT/PE

E the Number Needed to Treat (NNT) to prevent one DVT/PE is 100/1.5 = 67

Question 101

A committee is deciding whether a trial of a new treatment against an established treatment of a malignancy is ethical. Which one of the following would mean that the trial was ethically justifiable?

A the new treatment is thought to be better than the established treatment

B the established treatment is not a very effective treatment of the malignancy

C it is not certain which of the two treatments is best

D the established treatment is effective, but has a very high incidence of significant side effects

E the malignancy is very aggressive, with a median survival of 6 months with the established treatment

Question 102

If data are skewed, then they should be summarized in the form:

A mean and standard deviation

B median and range

C mean and range

D median and standard deviation

E mean and 95% confidence intervals

Question 103

The number needed to treat (NNT) is:

A 1 divided by absolute risk reduction

B 1 divided by relative risk reduction

C 1 divided by the p value

D 100 divided by relative risk reduction

E the same as the absolute risk reduction

Question 104

In a study of patients with myocardial infarction, the death rate of those given aspirin is 8%, compared with 10% in those not given aspirin. This means that the:

A relative risk of death after myocardial infarction is 1.25 in those given aspirin

B relative risk reduction produced by aspirin is 2%

C number needed to treat with aspirin to prevent one death is 8

D number needed to treat with aspirin to prevent one death is 10

E absolute risk reduction produced by aspirin is 2%

Question 105

To compare two groups of categorical data, e.g. dead/alive by drug/placebo, the correct test is:

A Student's t-test

B Analysis of variance (ANOVA)

C Wilcoxon rank-sum

D chi-squared

E p value

Pain relief and palliative care

G Nicola Rudd

Pain Relief and Palliative Care

Answers are on pp. 141–142.

Question 106

A 78-year-old woman with carcinoma of the ovary is admitted with a 4-day history of constipation associated with colicky abdominal pain and vomiting. Which two of the following would you do?

A prescribe a laxative and paracetamol
B order a plain abdominal radiograph
C prescribe oramorph and metoclopramide
D arrange an abdominal ultrasound
E give a stat dose of diamorphine
F prescribe hyoscine butylbromide and cyclizine orally
G seek a surgical opinion
H insert a nasogastric tube
I start a syringe driver with diamorphine and metoclopramide
J start a syringe driver with diamorphine and cyclizine

Question 107

A 58-year-old woman with metastatic renal cancer presents with severe right leg pain radiating from her buttock to her toes. A recent CT scan demonstrates epidural invasion at L1–L4. The pain is described as sharp, tingling and she has altered sensations in her lower leg. There has been little response to 20 mg bd of morphine. What two initial approaches should be tried to control her pain?

A arrange radiotherapy
B titrate morphine dose
C give intravenous bisphosphonate
D arrange urgent intrathecal analgaesia
E add in paracetamol
F ask a counsellor to talk with her
G add in amitriptyline or gabapentin
H change to fentanyl patch
I refer back to oncologist for further chemotherapy
J set up diamorphine syringe driver

Question 108

A 78-year-old woman with carcinoma of the ovary is admitted with colicky abdominal pain and vomiting. A plain abdominal radiograph shows multiple fluid levels and no stool. She is on diamorphine in a syringe driver, but the pain persists. What would be your preferred two immediate options?

A give diamorphine prn
B add a fentanyl patch
C increase the dose of diamorphine in the syringe driver
D give a stat dose of midazolam
E add hyoscine hydrobromide
F insert a nasogastric tube
G give diazepam PR
H add hyoscine butylbromide to the syringe driver
I add midazolam to the syringe driver
J organise an abdominal ultrasound

Question 109

You have decided to start a syringe driver on a dying patient whose symptoms were previously well controlled on oxycodone SR (OxyContin) 80 mg bd. What dose of diamorphine should you chose for your 24-hour syringe driver?

A 30 mg
B 60 mg
C 90 mg
D 110 mg
E 130 mg

Question 110

A 69-year-old man with disseminated colon cancer is admitted with vomiting. You want to prescribe an antiemetic, but he is terrified that he might develop constipation, which has been a considerable problem for him in the past. Which one of the following antiemetic drugs used in palliative care is not associated with constipation?

A ondansetron
B hyoscine
C cyclizine
D haloperidol
E levomepromazine

Question 111

A 54-year-old man with renal cell carcinoma and bone metastases is admitted with confusion and constipation.

He is on morphine sulphate continus MST 100 mg bd and a non-steroidal anti-inflammatory drug. How would you manage him?

A avoid intrusive investigations and treat symptoms as they arise

B stop opiates which may be the cause of his symptoms

C reduce opiates

D change opiates

E check serum calcium

Question 112

A 58-year-old woman with carcinoma of the ovary has been taking morphine sulphate continus (MST) 200 mg bd for 3 months. She presents with a 2-day history of twitching and drowsiness. Examination reveals her to be fluid overloaded and have pin point pupils. What is the most likely cause of her symptoms?

A acute renal failure

B morphine overdose

C renal failure leading to accumulation of morphine

D brain secondaries

E right sided cardiac failure

Question 113

A 58-year-old woman with metastatic carcinoma of the breast has good pain control on morphine sulphate continus MST 180mg bd. She is admitted with increasing weakness and has difficulty swallowing her tablets. It is therefore decided to convert her to a 24-hour diamorphine syringe driver. The correct dose of diamorphine is:

A 30 mg with 5 mg prn

B 60 mg with 10 mg prn

C 60 mg with 5 mg prn

D 120 mg with 10 mg prn

E 120 mg with 20 mg prn

Question 114

It has been decided that a patient should be changed from morphine sulphate continus MST 100 mg bd to the equivalent transdermal fentanyl dose. Choose the correct dose from those shown below:

A 125 µg/hr

B 25 µg/hr

C 100 µg/hr

D 50 µg/hr

E 75 µg/hr

Emergency medicine

C Andrew Eynon, Paul F Jenkins *(Editor)* and
Carole M Gavin

Emergency Medicine

Answers are on pp. 142–143.

Question 115

A 70-year-old man presents with a history of feeling faint on several occasions in the last month, although he has never collapsed. On examination his pulse is 40/min. His ECG is shown (see Figure 1). The diagnosis is:

A sinus bradycardia

B sick sinus syndrome

C 1st degree AV block

D 2nd degree AV block

E 3rd degree AV block

Question 116

A 48-year-old man presents with 48 hours of fever, rigors, breathlessness and bilateral pleuritic chest pain which came on as he thought that he was recovering from an attack of 'flu. He is very unwell, with cyanosis, pulse 120/min, respiratory rate 24/min and BP 100/60 mmHg. His chest radiograph is shown (see Figure 2). The diagnosis is:

A lobar pneumonia (right upper lobe)

B lobar pneumonia (right middle lobe)

C lobar pneumonia (right upper lobe) with left pneumothorax

D lobar pneumonia (right middle lobe) with left pneumothorax

E lobar pneumonia (right middle lobe) with loculated right pleural effusion

Question 117

You are walking onto a ward when you notice that a 78-year-old man has collapsed in his bed. Your first two actions should be:

A call the cardiac arrest team

B defibrillate (200 J)

C check that the situation is safe

D check responsiveness (shake and shout)

E check breathing (observe for movement of the chest)

F open airway (head tilt/chin lift)

G start chest compression

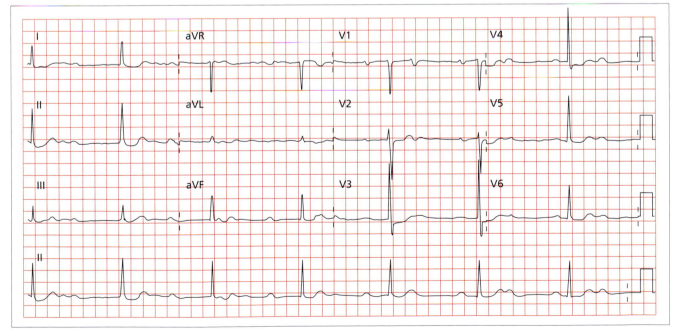

Fig. 1 Question 115.

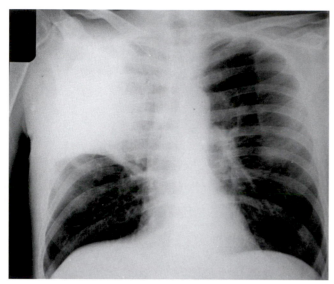

Fig. 2 Question 116.

H check for pulse (carotid)
I give precordial thump
J check for pulse (femoral)

Question 118

An elderly man is brought into the Accident and Emergency department by ambulance because he had been found wandering down his street early in the morning. He gives a fluent history of his past life, but is unable to explain what he had been doing. On examination he smells of alcohol. He has nystagmus and bilateral lateral gaze palsies. Which of the following statements is NOT correct?

A the lesions are in the mamillary bodies and thalamus
B his red cell transketolase is low
C examination of his pupils is normal
D all of his deficits will resolve with 3 days of parenteral thiamine
E a CT scan of his head is likely to be normal

Question 119

A 25-year-old woman presents to the Accident and Emergency department 1 hour after consuming 28×500 mg paracetamol tablets. Which of the following statements is true?

A if the INR is normal on a sample taken four hours from the time of ingestion, liver damage is unlikely to occur
B alcohol ingestion at the time of consumption of paracetamol is an indication for N-acetyl-cysteine treatment if paracetamol level at 4 hours exceeds the 'high-risk' line

C activated charcoal may be beneficial if given immediately
D onset of tinnitus may be an early symptom of liver failure
E deterioration in conscious level within the first 24 hours usually suggests hepatic encephalopathy

Question 120

A 50-year-old man presents with sudden onset shortness of breath and pleuritic chest pain. He has a CT pulmonary angiogram, which shows a large pulmonary embolus. Which of the following is NOT an indication for thrombolysis in this patient?

A cardiac arrest
B falling blood pressure
C D-dimer greater than 4000
D engorgement of neck veins
E right ventricular gallop

Question 121

An 18-year-old woman is admitted having deliberately taken a large overdose of her father's atenolol tablets. Which of the following statements is NOT true?

A dizziness is a common feature of beta-blocker overdose
B a temporary pacing wire may be required.
C atropine should not be given due to the risk of causing tachycardia
D glucagon is a useful therapy in the management of beta-blocker overdose
E paracetamol levels should be measured

Question 122

A 27-year-old woman develops difficulty breathing and her lips and tongue swell about five minutes after starting to eat a curry. She is brought to the Accident and Emergency department by ambulance. She is cyanosed and wheezing. Aside from high flow oxygen via a reservoir bag, which of the following treatments would be your top priority?

A hydrocortisone 200 mg intravenously
B chlorpheniramine 10 mg intravenously
C epinephrine (adrenaline)—0.5 ml of 1/1000 solution intravenously
D epinephrine (adrenaline)—0.5 ml of 1/1000 solution intramuscularly
E salbutamol 5 mg nebulized

Question 123

An 82-year-old man is admitted after a syncopal episode. His pulse rate is 40/min and ECG confirms complete

(3rd degree) heart block. His pulse slows to 24/min and he feels very faint. Whilst arrangements are being made for temporary pacing you give:

A adrenaline 0.5 mg intravenous bolus
B isoprenaline 50 mg intravenous bolus
C atropine 0.5 mg intravenous bolus
D atropine 5 mg intravenous bolus
E isoprenaline 500 mg intravenous bolus

Question 124
A 35-year-old woman presents 6 hours after a deliberate overdose of paracetamol. The paracetamol level at 6 hours is above the treatment line. Thirty minutes after starting an infusion of *N*-acetyl cysteine (NAC) she becomes flushed and hypotensive with a blood pressure of 80/55 mmHg. The infusion is stopped immediately and 500 ml IV 0.9% saline administered over 30 minutes. Which of the following is the correct ongoing management?

A IV chlorpheniramine and restart NAC infusion at lowest rate once symptoms resolved
B IV chlorpromazine and restart NAC infusion at lowest rate once symptoms resolved
C IV chlorpheniramine and give 2.5 g of oral methionine
D IV chlorpromazine and give 2.5 g of oral methionine
E withhold treatment and recheck paracetamol level at 12 hours

Infectious diseases

**Alec Bonington, Carolyn Hemsley,
Michael Jacobs, Paul Klenerman and
William Lynn** *(Editor)*

Infectious Diseases

Answers are on pp. 143–145.

Question 125

Figure 3 shows a swelling that developed 4 weeks after starting combination anti-retroviral therapy in an AIDS patient with a CD4 count of 20 cells/microlitre. Incision and drainage of an abscess was performed. What is the likely cause?

A mycobacterium avium intracellulare
B mycobacterium tuberculosis
C staphylococcus albus
D staphylococcus aureus
E lymphoma

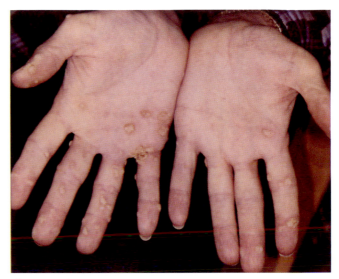

Fig. 4 Question 126.

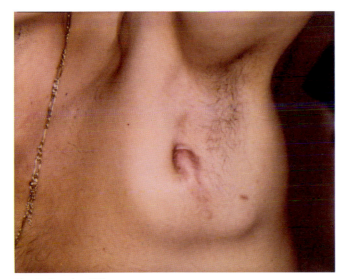

Fig. 3 Question 125.

D Epstein Barr virus
E molluscum contagiosum

Question 127

A 33-year-old man presents with abdominal pain 3 months after returning from a trip to India. Figure 5 shows a CT scan of his abdomen. What is the most likely cause of the abscess in his liver?

A tuberculosis
B pyogenic bacteria
C amoebiasis
D brucellosis
E hydatid

Question 126

A 40-year-old woman with chronic renal failure due to IgA nephropathy presents 3 years after a renal transplant with spots on her hands (see Figure 4). These have gradually increased in number over a period of 6 months. What is the cause?

A chicken pox
B papilloma virus
C cytomegalovirus

Question 128

A 20-year-old student becomes acutely unwell and is admitted on medical take with headache and fever. On examination he is hypotensive, but there are no focal signs. A year ago he went on a trekking holiday in southern Africa, but there is no more recent travel history. Figure 6 shows his blood film. What is the likely diagnosis?

A falciparum malaria
B vivax malaria

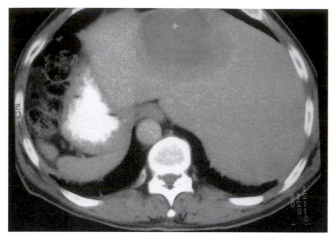

Fig. 5 Question 127.

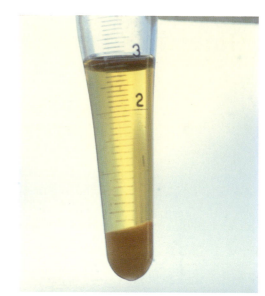

Fig. 7 Question 129.

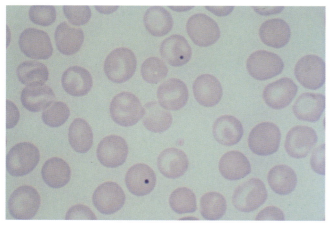

Fig. 6 Question 128.

Question 130

Figure 8 shows the eye of a 40-year-old woman presenting with a runny nose, fever and myalgia. What is the most likely diagnosis?

A streptococcal infection
B staphylococcal infection
C haemophilus infection
D varicella zoster infection
E adenovirus infection

C meningococcal septicaemia
D pneumococcal septicaemia
E dengue

Question 129

Figure 7 shows a serum sample from a 33-year-old woman presenting with arthritis and ankle swelling who is found to have proteinuria and abnormal liver function. What is the most likely diagnosis?

A rheumatoid arthritis
B systemic lupus erythematosus
C parvovirus infection
D hepatitis B infection
E hepatitis C infection

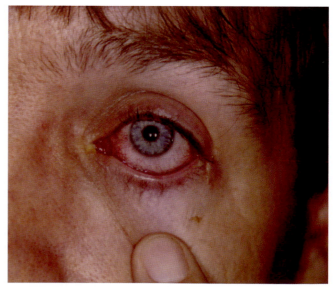

Fig. 8 Question 130.

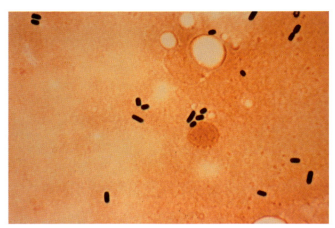

Fig. 9 Question 131.

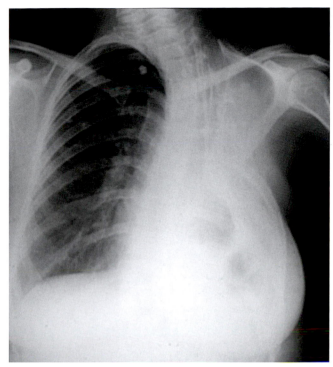

Fig. 10 Question 132.

Question 131

A 58-year-old man presents with fever and malaise. He is very unwell, with severe hypotension. He has an abscess on his foot. Figure 9 shows a Gram stain of material aspirated from this. What is the diagnosis?

A streptococcal infection
B staphylococcal infection
C infection with *Clostridium tetani*
D infection with *Clostridium perfringens*
E infection with *Neisseria meningitidis*

Question 132

A 74-year-old woman has developed a large inguinal hernia that is causing her distress. It has not proved possible to restrain this with a truss and she would like to have it corrected surgically. Her chest radiograph is shown (see Figure 10). What is the explanation?

A congenital kyphoscoliosis
B congenital kyphoscoliosis with left sided pleural effusion
C tuberculosis treated with thoracoplasty
D tuberculosis treated with plombage
E left sided pleural effusion

Question 133

A 65-year-old man with a history of controlled chronic myeloid leukaemia presents confused and unwell with a high fever but no other localizing signs of infection. Which combination of drugs would be the most appropriate treatment pending CSF analysis and blood culture results? (Select 2 options from this list)

A third generation cephalosporin
B high dose intravenous ampicillin
C high dose intravenous benzyl penicillin

D intravenous metronidazole
E oral aciclovir
F intravenous ciprofloxacin
G high dose intravenous flucloxacillin
H oral metronidazole
I intravenous vancomycin
J oral rifampicin

Question 134

You are called to see a 79-year-old man on the urology ward who has become unwell. He had a transurethral prostatectomy 6 hours ago and is now afebrile, vomiting, hypotensive and hypoxic. Preoperative investigations included a chest radiograph consistent with chronic obstructive airway disease, a CSU showing profuse growth of mixed coliforms and routine screening for methicillin-resistant *staphylococcus aureus* (MRSA) was positive. Blood tests showed mild renal impairment. Which two of the following are LEAST appropriate steps for immediate management?

A oxygen administration via a facemask
B fluid resuscitation
C commencement of oral ciprofloxacin 500 mg b.d.
D commencement of intravenous cefuroxime 1.5 g t.d.s. with addition of 500 mg t.d.s. metronidazole

E commencement of intravenous cefuroxime 1.5 g t.d.s. with addition of vancomycin 750 mg b.d.

F taking an ECG

G repeating a chest radiograph

H taking blood cultures

I placement on regular observations

J taking blood gases

Question 135

A 32-year-old woman who might be pregnant has recently returned from Africa. She is febrile and drowsy with a *Plasmodium falciparum* malaria parasite count of 1%, haemoglobin of 9.8 g/dl, platelets of 20×10^9/l, creatinine of 200 μmol/l and mild jaundice. Which two of the following are essential parts of her management?

A CT of her head

B platelet transfusion

C blood glucose monitoring

D exchange transfusion

E dialysis

F liver ultrasound

G prophylactic phenobarbitone

H steroids

I antimalarial treatment given intravenously

J antibiotic cover

Question 136

A 48-year-old man presents with a 5-day history of fever and cough. He has no significant past medical history but is very unwell. His chest radiograph shows patchy shadowing, mainly in the right lower lobe. What two antibiotic regimen from the list below would it be most appropriate to give him?

A co-trimoxazole 120 mg/kg daily in 2–4 divided doses

B ciprofloxacin 400 mg 12-hourly intravenously

C erythromycin 1 g 6-hourly intravenously

D clarithromycin 250 mg 8-hourly orally

E ciprofloxacin 500 mg 12-hourly orally

F erythromycin 500 mg 6-hourly intravenously

G benzylpenicillin 1.2–2.4 g 6-hourly intravenously

H rifampicin 600 mg 12-hourly intravenously

I amoxicillin 250 mg 8-hourly orally

J cefotaxime 1 g 8-hourly intravenously

Question 137

A 40-year-old woman, recently returned from a 2-month trip to India, presents with a week's history of fever, malaise, myalgia and headache. There are no abnormal findings on examination. A full blood count shows Hb 13.6 g/dl, WCC 14.2×10^9/l (neutrophils 12.4×10^9/l), platelets 148×10^9/l. A malaria film is negative. Which one of the following would be UNLIKELY?

A rickettsial disease

B amoebic liver abscess

C leptospirosis

D urinary tract infection

E sepsis from pyodermic insect bites

Question 138

A 30-year-old man, recently returned from trekking in Nepal, presents with a 6-day history of bloody diarrhoea with abdominal cramps but no fevers. He has taken some antibiotics, obtained in Nepal, with little effect. Which one of the following would be an UNLIKELY cause?

A *Entamoeba histolytica*

B *Trichuris*

C acute schistosomiasis

D ulcerative colitis

E *Clostridium difficile* colitis

Question 139

Two days after returning from a 1-week trip around Thailand, a 25-year-old woman presents with sudden onset of fever, headache and severe myalgia. Three days after her symptoms started she develops a generalized erythematous rash. Her Hb is 12g/dl, WCC 2.1×10^9/l and platelets 65×10^9/l. What is the most likely diagnosis?

A *Plasmodium vivax* malaria

B typhoid fever

C paratyphoid fever

D dengue fever

E tick-borne encephalitis

Dermatology

Karen Harman *(Editor)*, Graham Ogg and
Natalie M Stone

Dermatology

Answers are on pp. 145–146.

Question 140

Figure 11 shows a 24-year-old woman who developed an acute papular rash on her trunk and proximal limbs. She was not unwell or feverish, but had suffered from a sore throat one week previously. On close inspection, the surface of the red papules was scaly. What is the likely diagnosis?

A chickenpox
B eczema herpeticum
C psoriasis
D pemphigoid
E pemphigus

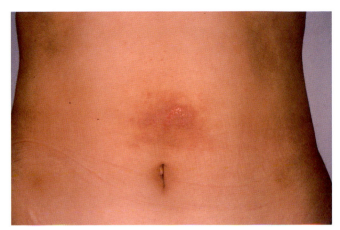

Fig. 12 Question 141.

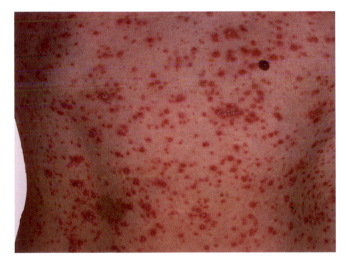

Fig. 11 Question 140.

Question 141

Figure 12 shows a 19-year-old woman who developed a rash on her abdomen. What is the likely diagnosis?

A erythema multiforme
B psoriasis
C irritant contact dermatitis
D allergic contact dermatitis
E atopic eczema

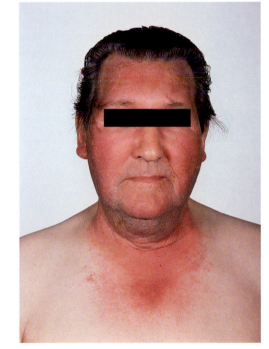

Fig. 13 Question 142.

Question 142

A 64-year-old man developed a scaly, itchy rash on his face and hands (see Figure 13). What is the likely diagnosis?

A psoriasis
B systemic lupus erythematosus
C irritant contact dermatitis
D allergic contact dermatitis
E photosensitive eczema

Question 143

A 40-year-old Indian man presents with mouth ulcers, a sore penis and ulcers on the skin. Which would be the two most helpful investigations in reaching a diagnosis?
A patch tests
B direct immunofluorescence
C pathergy test
D autoantibody screen
E skin prick tests
F skin biopsy
G skin scrapings
H skin swab
I Tzanck smear
J IgE level

Question 144

A 28-year-old man presents with a 3-month history of the daily development of itchy erythematous weals each of which lasts several hours and then resolve without scaling. Which two of the following statements are true of chronic urticaria?
A with a careful history, it is possible to identify the trigger in virtually all cases
B it is thought to be predominantly IgE-mediated
C it is associated with internal malignancy

D it can be associated with systemic lupus erythematous (SLE)
E vasculitic changes are often seen on biopsy
F H1-antagonists provide an important therapeutic option
G H2-antagonists have no significant role in therapy
H most patients have disease lasting longer than 10 years
I essential investigations would include a chest radiograph
J non-steroidal anti-inflammatory drugs are often useful therapeutically

Question 145

A 60-year-old woman with rheumatoid arthritis presents with a rapidly enlarging, painful, sloughy leg ulcer on the anterior shin. Doppler examination is normal. There has been no improvement with dressings and bandages. What would be the most appropriate next step in management?
A referral to surgeons for debridement
B referral to surgeons for grafting
C maggot therapy
D compression
E immunosupression

Question 146

A 50-year-old man presents with hair loss. Examination reveals patches of scarring alopecia with surrounding inflammation. Which is the most likely diagnosis?
A lichen planopilaris
B androgenetic alopecia
C alopecia areata
D traction alopecia
E trichotillomania

Haematology

Kristian M Bowles, David W Galvani *(Editor)*
and Bronwen E Shaw

Haematology

Answers are on pp. 146–148.

Question 147

A 77-year-old woman is admitted to hospital having 'gone off her legs'. She says that she has felt tired for many months. She looks pale, but examination is otherwise unremarkable. Her blood count shows haemoglobin 6.7 g/dl, white cell count 4.3×10^9/l and platelets 76×10^9/l. Figure 14 shows her blood film. The most likely diagnosis is:

A myelodysplasia
B B12 deficiency
C iron deficiency
D acute myeloid leukaemia
E folate deficiency

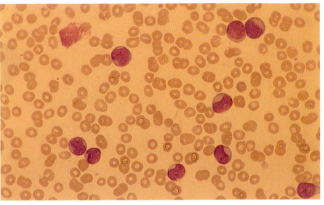

Fig. 15 Question 148.

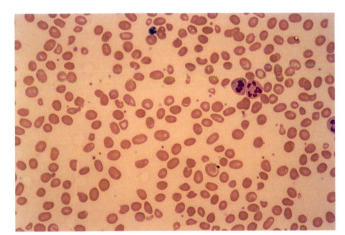

Fig. 14 Question 147.

Question 148

A 63-year-old man is admitted to hospital with pneumonia. His blood count shows haemoglobin 9.2 g/dl, white cell count 14×10^9/l and platelets 23×10^9/l. Figure 15 shows his blood film. The most likely diagnosis is:

A myelodysplasia
B acute lymphocytic leukaemia
C acute myeloid leukaemia
D chronic lymphocytic leukaemia
E myeloma

Question 149

A 65-year-old man has received chemotherapy for acute myeloblastic leukaemia through his Hickman line. His left arm has become swollen and uncomfortable (see Figure 16). The key investigation to establish the diagnosis is:

A blood D-dimer
B chest radiograph
C ultrasound examination of venous supply of the arm
D contrast imaging of venous supply of the arm (venography)
E lung ventilation/perfusion scan

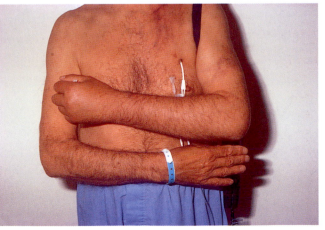

Fig. 16 Question 149.

Question 150

A 30-year-old man is admitted to hospital with a history of a few days of fever, malaise and breathlessness. His wife has had similar symptoms. His blood count is reported as follows: haemoglobin 9.7 g/dl, mean corpuscular volume 121 fl, white cell count 12.1×10^9/l and platelets 278×10^9/l. Figure 17 shows his blood film. The most likely diagnosis is:

A B12 deficiency, with probable viral illness
B folate deficiency, with probable viral illness
C acute myeloid leukaemia
D myeloma
E mycoplasma infection

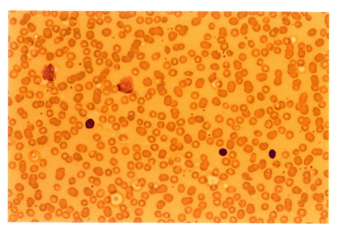

Fig. 18 Question 151.

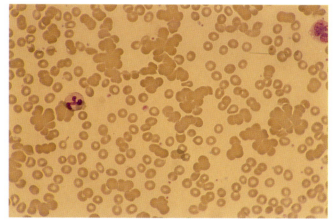

Fig. 17 Question 150.

Question 151

A 74-year-old man is admitted for repair of an inguinal hernia. He has had a recent cold, but is otherwise well. A routine full blood count is as follows: haemoglobin 14.2 g/dl, white cell count 25×10^9/l and platelets 374×10^9/l. Figure 18 shows his blood film. What is the diagnosis?

A normal
B intercurrent infection
C acute myeloid leukaemia
D chronic myeloid leukaemia
E chronic lymphatic leukaemia

Question 152

A 48-year-old man wakes up noticing a generalised rash over his body. A week previously he had developed a 'flu-like' illness. His full blood count showed Hb 12.4 g/dl, WBC 8×10^9/l and platelets 2×10^9/l. A bone marrow showed no atypical cells but adequate megakaryocytes. Which two of the following treatments are options in an actively bleeding patient with immune thrombocytopenic purpura (ITP)?

A peripheral vasoconstrictors
B corticosteroids
C fresh frozen plasma (FFP) infusion
D low molecular weight heparin
E intravenous immunoglobulin infusion
F cautery and laser diathermy of bleeding point
G transfusion of single unit of matched platelets
H topical fibrin glue
I hydroxyurea
J leucocyte infusion

Question 153

A 22-year-old woman has had heavy periods ever since she can remember, certainly for many years, and is now iron deficient. What two conditions must be considered?

A haemophilia
B coeliac disease
C disseminated intravascular coagulation (DIC)
D chronic liver disease
E idiopathic thrombocytopenic purpura (ITP)
F hypothyroidism
G Cushing's syndrome
H Von Willebrand's disease
I chronic renal failure
J hyperthyroidism

Question 154

A 47-year-old decorator has hereditary spherocytosis. His Hb is 11 g/dl, MCV 89 fl, bilirubin 23 μmol/l. He copes with his job but asks if splenectomy may help. Which two of the following statements are correct?

A splenectomy is without serious consequences
B folic acid replacement can usually obviate the need for splenectomy
C splenectomy is indicated for symptomatic anaemia
D splenectomy should always be followed by B12 replacement
E splenectomy does not require vaccination in adults
F splenectomy should be routinely performed at the age of 7 years
G splenectomy is indicated for splenomegaly in spherocytosis
H splenectomy is indicated for uncompensated haemolysis
I splenectomy always improves the Hb level
J splenectomy reduces the number of circulating spherocytes

Question 155

You are given a blood count by the gastroenterology secretary. It is from a 67-year-old woman in last week's clinic. It shows Hb 8.5 g/dl, MCV 122 fl, platelets 98×10^9/l, neutrophils 1.2×10^9/l. Your next two steps should be to:
A organise a Schilling test
B phone the general practitioner to ask him/her to check B12 and folate levels
C ask the haematology laboratory to check the reticulocyte count on the sample
D phone the consultant gastroenterologist
E check to see what the blood film showed
F arrange for the patient to commence intramuscular vitamin B12
G phone the consultant haematologist
H arrange for the patient to commence oral folate
I ask the haematology laboratory to check a Coomb's test
J make a note for the problem to be reviewed at the next clinic visit

Question 156

The use of anti-D immunoglobulin has all but wiped out cases of haemolytic disease of the newborn in this country. Not all women need to be given anti-D and it should not be given to women who do not need it. Which two of the following women would require further testing and anti-D after delivery? For the scenarios below F = father's blood group, M = mother's blood group, B = baby's blood group.
A M = A RhD -ve, F = O RhD -ve, B = O RhD -ve
B M = AB RhD +ve, F = B RhD -ve, B = O RhD -ve
C M = B RhD -ve, F = B RhD +ve, B = O RhD +ve
D M = O RhD +ve, F = B RhD -ve, B = O RhD +ve
E M = O Rh -ve, F = AB RhD +ve, B = B RhD -ve
F M = B RhD +ve, F = B RhD -ve, B = AB RhD +ve
G M = AB RhD +ve, F = AB RhD -ve, B = ARhD +ve
H M = O RhD -ve, F = B RhD -ve, B = O RhD -ve
I M = O RhD -ve, F = B RhD +ve, B = ORhD +ve
J M = O RhD +ve, F = O RhD +ve, B = ORhD -ve

Question 157

A 45-year-old man, previously well, receives a unit of blood on a surgical ward. Shortly after the transfusion commences you are bleeped and told that he has had a severe reaction to the blood. Which two of the following are the most common causes of this scenario?
A incorrect blood unit being given (i.e. for another patient)
B bacterial infection of blood
C reaction to HLA antibodies
D circulatory overload
E incorrect sample sent to blood bank (resulting in the incorrect blood for the patient)
F allergic reaction to white cells
G graft versus host disease
H reaction to plasma proteins
I immune sensitization
J allergic reaction to platelets

Question 158

A young man presents to the Accident and Emergency department with a history of a febrile illness. His full blood count reveals lymphopenia. Which two of the following are most likely to explain this finding?
A infectious mononucleosis
B HIV infection
C lymphoma
D tuberculosis
E malaria
F acute leukaemia
G food poisoning
H bacterial pneumonia
I influenza
J exercise

Question 159

A 16-year-old boy has been diagnosed with acute lymphoblastic leukaemia (ALL). His white cell count is 10×10^9/l, platelet count 100×10^9/l and Hb 14 g/dl at diagnosis. Which one of these factors is associated with a better outcome?

A his age
B his gender
C his haemoglobin
D his white cell count
E his platelet count

Question 160

A 68-year-old woman has had chronic lymphocytic leukaemia (CLL) for 4 years without marrow failure or any need for medication. At follow up, her haemoglobin has dropped to 7.8 g/dl, with other tests showing mean corpuscular volume (MCV) 122 fl, platelets 211×10^9/l, lymphocytes 43×10^9/l, reticulocyte count 12%. Which test is most likely to give you the correct diagnosis?

A serum B12 level
B Coombs test
C marrow aspirate
D red cell folate level
E serum ferritin level

Question 161

A 71-year-old man was treated with fludarabine for Waldenström's macroglobulinaemia. His IgM band fell from 36 g/l to a plateau of 5 g/l and he was stable for 5 years before suddenly presenting with Hb 6.7 g/dl, platelets 79×10^9/l, creatinine 130 μmol/l and plasma viscosity 2.5 mPa/s (normal range 1.5–1.75). During blood transfusion he developed a tachycardia and chest pain and was transferred to the Coronary Care Unit. The next day results showed Hb 7 g/dl, Coombs' test positive, creatinine 377 μmol/l. What is the most likely diagnosis?

A renal failure due to hyperviscosity
B cardiac ischaemia due to anaemia
C fludarabine induced haemolysis
D relapse of Waldenström's with haemolytic transfusion reaction
E transformation to acute leukaemia

Question 162

A 78-year-old woman presents with a 3-month history of worsening back pain. Her full blood count reveals haemoglobin 10.2 g/dl and there are rouleaux on the blood film. She has moderately impaired renal function. You suspect myeloma but dipstick testing of her urine is negative for protein and serum electrophoresis fails to demonstrate a monoclonal band. Which one of the following statements is true?

A she does not have myeloma
B polymyalgia rheumatica is the most likely diagnosis
C she may have myeloma that produces only free light chains
D bone pain is an unusual presentation of myeloma
E negative protein on dipstick testing of urine rules out the presence of Bence-Jones protein

Question 163

A 26-year-old woman attends the warfarin clinic that you are running. She is quite well with no evidence of bleeding or increased bruising. She is on no other medication. Unexpectedly her INR is 7.5. What is the correct course of action?

A administer 10 mg of Vitamin K intravenously
B administer 10 mg of Vitamin K orally
C admit for fresh frozen plasma (FFP) infusion
D stop warfarin and recheck her INR in 3 days
E admit overnight for observation

Oncology

Mark Bower *(Editor)* and Graham G Dark

Oncology

Answers are on pp. 148–149.

Question 164

This technetium-99 pyrophosphate bone scan (Figure 19) from a patient with known prostate cancer shows:

A normal appearances

B multiple bone metastases

C multiple bone metastases and non-functioning left kidney

D multiple bone metastases and splenic metastases

E multiple bone metastases and hepatic metastases

Question 165

Figure 20 is a chest radiograph of a 60-year-old man treated 10 years previously for non-small cell lung cancer. The appearances are most likely to be due to:

A recurrent tumour

B post-radiation fibrosis

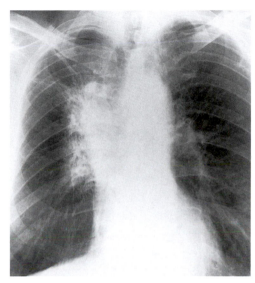

Fig. 20 Question 165.

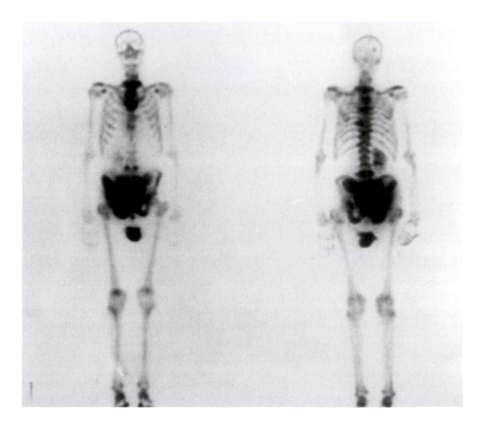

Fig. 19 Question 164.

C lung fibrosis secondary to chemotherapy
D secondary lymphoma
E tuberculosis

Question 166
A 68-year-old man presents with a 3-week history of increasing confusion and headaches. A CT scan of the brain reveals multiple metastatic lesions. Which are the two most likely primary sites?
A renal carcinoma
B squamous carcinoma of the lung
C prostate
D melanoma
E rectum
F small cell lung cancer
G large cell lung cancer
H oesophageal adenocarcinoma
I stomach
J oral cavity

Question 167
A 43-year-old woman presents with a mass in her axilla. Examination is otherwise unremarkable. Biopsy of the mass reveals poorly differentiated carcinoma. A 38-year-old woman presents with ascites and is found to have peritoneal carcinomatosis, but again no primary tumour can be identified. For which two of the following unknown primary tumours can treatment be effective?
A liver
B kidney
C melanoma
D breast
E colon
F lung
G pancreas
H oesophagus
I ovary
J stomach

Question 168
On auscultation of the heart, a patient with known carcinoid syndrome is found to have a murmur. Which two cardiac valvular lesions are most likely to occur in a patient with this condition?
A mitral stenosis
B mitral regurgitation
C tricuspid stenosis
D tricuspid regurgitation

E pulmonary stenosis
F pulmonary regurgitation
G aortic stenosis
H aortic regurgitation
I mitral stenosis with aortic regurgitation
J pulmonary stenosis with aortic regurgitation

Question 169
A general practitioner rings you about an 82-year-old man with multiple myeloma. The patient has recently started to experience unsteadiness when walking and has fallen several times in the last 24 hours. What advice would you give?
A send the patient to hospital as an emergency
B arrange to see the patient within the next few days in the next available clinic slot.
C arrange a CT or MRI brain scan.
D ask the general practitioner to exclude an underlying infection
E start the patient on high-dose steroids

Question 170
A 62-year-old man presents with altered bowel habit and has positive faecal occult bloods. Colonoscopy reveals a tight sigmoid adenocarcinoma. A staging CT scan shows two metastases in the left lobe of the liver. The initial treatment plan should be:
A chemotherapy prior to surgery
B left hemicolectomy and palliative chemotherapy
C chemo-radiotherapy to primary tumour, then continued palliative chemotherapy
D left hemicolectomy then consideration of liver resection
E palliative chemotherapy alone

Question 171
A 30-year-old man presents to his primary care physician with right leg pain of one year's duration. The pain is worse at night but is fully relieved by aspirin. A plain radiograph reveals a focally sclerotic expanded area of the tibial cortex, without overlying soft tissue or periosteal abnormalities. A radiolucent nidus is visible in the centre of the focal area of sclerosis. Radionuclide bone scintigraphy reveals a very prominent focal uptake of the radiotracer in the same region. What is the most likely diagnosis?
A osteoid osteoma
B stress fracture
C metastatic deposit

D trauma

E osteogenic sarcoma

Question 172

A 63-year-old woman presents with one episode of haemoptysis. She had been treated for node-positive, oestrogen-receptor positive left breast cancer four years previously with wide local excision and axillary dissection, adjuvant anthracycline chemotherapy, radiotherapy and tamoxifen, which she is still taking. Her chest radiograph reveals a left hilar lesion, confirmed on CT scan that is otherwise clear. Which of the following is appropriate initial management?

A withdraw tamoxifen and await tamoxifen withdrawal response

B commence second line hormone therapy with anastrazole

C positron emission tomography (PET) scan

D palliative chemotherapy with a taxane

E bronchoscopy and biopsy

Question 173

A 35-year-old woman presents with a 1 cm diameter lump in her left breast, which needle biopsy reveals to be invasive ductal carcinoma. What should her initial treatment be?

A wide local excision and axillary node sampling followed by adjuvant breast radiotherapy in all cases

B wide local excision and axillary node sampling followed by adjuvant breast radiotherapy if there is histological spread to the axillary nodes

C mastectomy and axillary node sampling followed by adjuvant breast radiotherapy in all cases

D mastectomy and axillary node sampling followed by adjuvant chemotherapy if there is histological spread to the axillary nodes

E wide local excision and axillary node sampling followed by adjuvant breast radiotherapy and adjuvant chemotherapy if there is histological spread to the axillary nodes

Cardiology

Peter E Glennon, Catherine EG Head,
Paul R Roberts *(Editor)* and
Hamish A Walker

Cardiology

Answers are on pp. 149–150.

Question 174

A 67-year-old man presents with chest pain that came on suddenly while he was lying in bed. It radiated to the left shoulder, and he felt sweaty and nauseated. His past medical history was notable for duodenal ulceration, 20 years previously, and hypertension, for which he took bendrofluazide as his only regular medication. On examination he looked unwell, with pulse 110/min (regular), BP 120/60 mmHg in both arms, and jugular venous pressure elevated 5 cm. On auscultation of the heart he had a soft pericardial rub and a short early diastolic murmur. His chest radiograph is shown (Figure 21). What is the most likely diagnosis?

A myocardial infarction
B pericarditis
C aortic dissection
D pulmonary embolus
E perforated duodenal ulcer

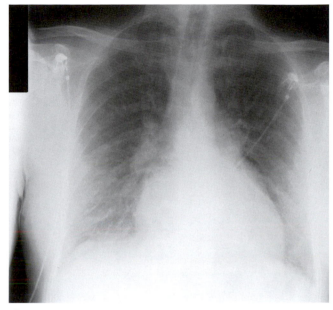

Fig. 22 Question 175.

Question 175

A 68-year-old man presents on the emergency medical take with breathlessness. His chest radiograph is shown (see Figure 22). Which is the best description of the radiograph?

A normal
B pulmonary oedema
C pulmonary oedema and cardiomegaly
D pulmonary oedema and cardiomegaly with enlarged right ventricle
E pulmonary oedema and cardiomegaly with enlarged left atrium

Question 176

A 70-year-old man, who is known to have ischaemic heart disease and has had short-lived episodes of atrial fibrillation in the past, presents with 48 hours of fatigue and breathlessness. He is not very ill, but his pulse is 150/min in atrial fibrillation. Which two drugs would be most appropriate to achieve 'chemical cardioversion'?

A digoxin
B quinidine

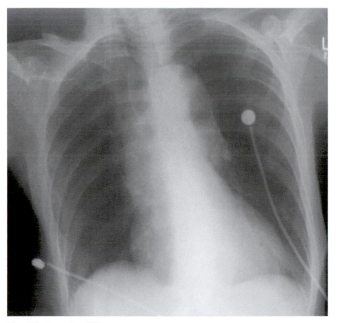

Fig. 21 Question 174.

C procainamide

D disopyramide

E sotalol

F atenolol

G propanolol

H verapamil

I amiodarone

J diltiazem

Question 177

A 45-year-old man is referred by his general practitioner with palpitations. He has no other associated symptoms and specifically he is not presyncopal. Holter monitoring has demonstrated short non-sustained runs of a mono-morphic broad complex tachycardia. Which two of the following are the most likely arrhythmias?

A sinus tachycardia

B atrial fibrillation with intermittent rate associated bundle branch block

C right ventricular outflow tract tachycardia

D atrial flutter with one to one conduction

E tachycardia associated with Wolff-Parkinson-White syndrome

F ischaemic ventricular tachycardia

G atrioventricular nodal reentry tachycardia

H ventricular fibrillation

I torsades de pointes

J atrioventricular reentry tachycardia

Question 178

You find a middle aged man on a path in a park. He has no pulse and is not breathing. What is the appropriate next step:

A give two rescue breaths and initiate CPR at a ratio of 5 compressions to 2 breaths

B give two rescue breaths and initiate CPR at a ratio of 15 compressions to 2 breaths

C give a precordial thump

D give two rescue breaths and go for help

E go to call 999 (emergency services) immediately

Question 179

A 70-year-old man with a past history of anterior myo-cardial infarction presents with syncope and ventricular tachycardia (VT). Angiography reveals that the left anter-ior descending (LAD) artery is occluded and there is poor left ventricular function. Thallium (nuclear) imag-ing reveals a fixed anterior defect with no evidence of reversible ischaemia. What would be the optimal thera-peutic strategy?

A amiodarone

B coronary artery bypass grafting and amiodarone

C implantable cardioverter defibrillator (ICD)

D implantable cardioverter defibrillator and beta-blocker

E percutaneous angioplasty to the LAD

Question 180

A 60-year-old woman presents with recurrent syncope; ECG reveals complete heart block. She is scheduled for a pacemaker. Which of the following pacemakers would be most appropriate?

A AOO

B DDD

C implantable cardioverter defibrillator (dual chamber)

D VVI

E VVIR

Question 181

A 70-year-old man is investigated for deteriorating angi-nal symptoms. Echo confirms a stenotic aortic valve with peak gradient 80 mmHg. Angiography demonstrates a discrete severe stenosis in his left anterior descending artery (LAD). Which would be the optimal treatment?

A aortic valve replacement

B aortic valve replacement and internal mammary artery graft to the LAD

C beta-blocker, aspirin, statin and review

D percutaneous coronary angioplasty to the LAD

E percutaneous aortic valvotomy and coronary angio-plasty to the LAD

Question 182

A 50-year-old man presents 3 months after mitral valve re-placement (metallic) with increasing shortness of breath, fever and weight loss. Clinically he is in pulmonary oedema. Transoesophageal echo (TOE) confirms severe paravalvular mitral regurgitation. The first blood culture is positive for *Staph epidermidis*. Which is the optimal therapeutic approach?

A intravenous antibiotics for 4 weeks and then repeat TOE

B oral antibiotics for 4 weeks and angiotensin-converting enzyme (ACE)—inhibitor

C start intravenous antibiotics and urgent re-do mitral valve replacement—bioprosthetic

D start intravenous antibiotics and urgent re-do mitral valve replacement—metallic
E withold antibiotics and repeat 3 sets of blood cultures

Question 183
A 32-year-old woman has been referred to you by her doctor, after complaining of syncope and breathlessness. Her sister died suddenly in her 20s. Clinically she has loud pulmonary second heart sound. What is the most likely diagnosis?
A aortic stenosis
B mitral stenosis
C tricuspid regurgitation
D primary pulmonary hypertension
E aortic regurgitation

Respiratory medicine

Praveen Bhatia, Michael I Polkey *(Editor)*
and Veronica LC White

Respiratory Medicine

Answers are on pp. 150–151.

Question 184

A 28-year-old man presents with breathlessness. He appears anxious, but physical examination is otherwise normal. His chest radiograph is shown (Figure 23). The diagnosis is:

A normal chest radiograph

B pulmonary oligaemia suggesting pulmonary embolism

C pneumothorax

D left lower lobe collapse

E right lower lobe collapse

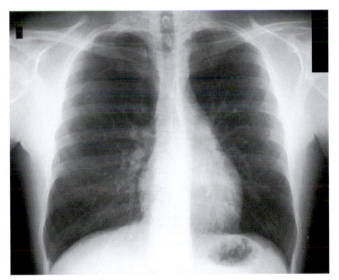

Fig. 23 Question 184.

Question 185

A 52-year-old woman presents with breathlessness that has been getting gradually worse for a couple of months. She smokes 10 cigarettes per day, which she has done for many years, has long-standing atrial fibrillation (AF), presumed ischaemic in origin, and takes furosemide, amiodarone, aspirin and atorvastatin as regular medications. On examination her pulse is 80/min (AF), blood pressure 120/80 mmHg, jugular venous pressure elevated 3 cm above the sternal angle and there are fine inspiratory crackles to mid zones bilaterally. Heart sounds are normal, and she does not have peripheral oedema. Her chest radiograph is shown (Figure 24). What is the most likely diagnosis?

A interstitial lung disease

B pulmonary oedema

C chronic pulmonary embolism

D chronic obstructive pulmonary disease

E late onset asthma

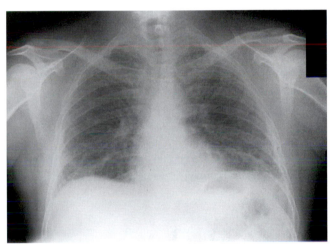

Fig. 24 Question 185.

Question 186

A 35-year-old man presents with a first episode of haemoptysis. He has felt a bit feverish for the last few days, but has not had sweats or rigors. He is generally fit and well and gives no history of previous respiratory problems. On examination his temperature is 37.8°C and his chest is clear. Which two of the following are the most likely diagnoses?

A pulmonary tuberculosis

B bronchiectasis

C pneumonia

D lung cancer

E benign bronchial tumour

F pulmonary arteriovenous malformation

G asthma

81

H chronic obstructive pulmonary disease
I   Goodpasture's syndrome
J   pulmonary embolism

Question 187

A 27-year-old woman with asthma is admitted with an acute attack. Her symptoms started around 8.00 am, but by 10.00 am she was so unwell that she needed admission to hospital. Shortly after arriving at the Accident and Emergency department she was transferred to the Intensive Care Unit. Similar incidents had occurred twice in the past. Which two of the following statements regarding near fatal asthma are correct?

A previous severe asthma attacks are a risk factor
B the short time lag between the start of symptoms and hospital admission is a risk factor
C females are especially at risk
D the risk increases in obese patients
E family history of asthma is common
F allergy to peanut is commoner in patients with near fatal asthma
G near fatal asthma occurs more frequently during the winter season
H long acting beta-2 agonists are beneficial in preventing asthma attacks
I   childhood eczema is a risk factor
J   parental smoking is a risk factor.

Question 188

A 37-year-old man with asthma comes to your clinic. His current medication consists of a low dose of inhaled corticosteroids and inhaled short-acting beta-2 agonist that he takes, on average, three to four times a day. What would you do?

A advise him to continue with his current medication
B commence a high dose of inhaled corticosteroid
C add an inhaled long-acting beta-2 agonist
D add a leucotriene receptor antagonist
E add a long-acting anticholinergic

Question 189

A 43-year-old woman with long-standing asthma is admitted with an exacerbation. She is cyanosed and unable to speak more than three words at a time. She is using her accessory muscles, chest expansion is reduced but the same on both sides, and a wheeze can be heard bilaterally. Which one of the following is the best initial treatment?

A maximum inspired oxygen by face mask; nebulised salbutamol (5 mg) driven by oxygen
B nebulised salbutamol (5 mg) driven by air
C nebulised salbutamol (50 mg) driven by oxygen
D oxygen 35% by face mask; nebulised salbutamol (10 mg) driven by 35% oxygen
E maximum inspired oxygen by face mask; decompress both sides of the chest by inserting venflons into the second intercostal spaces in the mid-clavicular line bilaterally.

Question 190

A 74-year-old man is treated in hospital for exacerbation of chronic obstructive pulmonary disease (COPD). His condition improves significantly and he is keen to go home. His repeated arterial blood gas (ABG) analysis (on air) shows a pH of 7.35, pCO_2 of 4.5 kPa, pO_2 of 7.1 kPa, HCO_3 of 26 mmol/L. What action would be most appropriate?

A prescribe the patient an oxygen cylinder on discharge
B discharge the patient once his ABG analysis returns to normal
C request an oxygen concentrator and discharge the patient once an oxygen concentrator is fitted
D discharge the patient and arrange a follow up in 6 weeks' time with a repeated ABG
E discharge the patient and advise a follow up by his GP

Question 191

A 58-year-old man, a smoker for many years despite repeated advice that he should stop, has chronic obstructive pulmonary disease (COPD) that is increasingly limiting his exercise capacity. You wish to conduct a trial of steroid therapy. Which of the following is the correct way of giving oral prednisolone and interpreting the outcome?

A 60 mg daily for 4 weeks, regarding a clear statement of subjective improvement by the patient as a positive response
B 10 mg daily for 2 weeks, regarding a clear statement of subjective improvement by the patient as a positive response if accompanied by a rise in FEV1
C 60 mg daily for 4 weeks, regarding a clear statement of subjective improvement by the patient as a positive response if accompanied by a rise in FEV1 of >10%
D 30 mg daily for 2 weeks, regarding an increase in FEV1 of >10% and >200 ml as a positive response
E 30 mg daily for 2 weeks, regarding a clear statement of subjective improvement by the patient as a positive response

Question 192

A 24-year-old man presents with fever, breathlessness, cough and sputum production. His only medical history of note is long-standing heavy alcohol consumption, but he had no respiratory complaint whatever until 6 weeks ago when he developed breathing difficulty with high fever and rigors. He was given antibiotics by his general practitioner and began to improve, but this improvement has not been sustained. The most likely diagnosis is:

A lung abscess

B bronchiectasis

C chronic obstructive pulmonary disease (COPD)

D asthma precipitated by chest infection

E empyema

Question 193

A 40-year-old woman, generally fit and well, is admitted with malaise and fever. Four weeks previously she had suffered a chest infection for which she was given a course of oral antibiotics. She felt better initially, but never recovered fully and is now getting worse. Her chest radiograph shows a right-sided pleural effusion. The most likely diagnosis is:

A connective tissue disorder

B lung cancer

C tuberculosis

D pulmonary embolism

E pneumonia with effusion/empyema

Gastroenterology and hepatology

Jane D Collier *(Editor)*, John M Hebden,
Satish Keshav and Jeremy Shearman

Gastroenterology and Hepatology

Answers are on pp. 152–154.

Question 194

A 48-year-old woman with no significant past medical history presents with abdominal pain. She has had diarrhoea for 4 weeks, recently up to 8 times per day. This was initially associated with griping abdominal pain, but over the last 24 hrs this has become worse, leading to her being sent to the Medical Admissions Unit. Her abdominal X-ray is shown (see Figure 25). What does the radiograph show?

A toxic megacolon
B constipation
C small bowel obstruction
D perforated viscus
E normal appearance

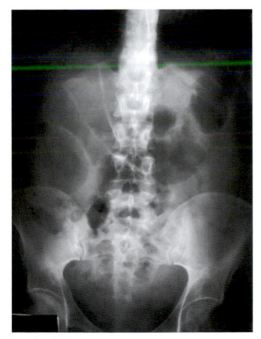

Fig. 25 Question 194.

Question 195

A 68-year-old Indian man, recently returned from a two month visit to his family in India, presents with alteration in bowel habit. Sometimes the bowels are loose, some- times constipated, and he has occasionally seen blood mixed in with the motions. His barium enema is shown (see Figure 26). What is the likely diagnosis?

A infective colitis
B ulcerative colitis
C Crohn's disease
D colonic carcinoma
E traveller's diarrhoea

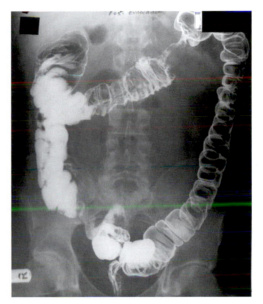

Fig. 26 Question 195.

Question 196

A 36-year-old ex-intravenous drug user is HCV-RNA positive with persistently elevated transaminases and has evidence of moderate to severe inflammation on liver biopsy. Which two of the following drugs may be used in her treatment?

A amantadine
B lobucavir
C lamivudine
D beta-interferon
E ribavirin
F anti-TNF-alpha antibodies
G ganciclovir
H alpha-interferon

I famciclovir

J aciclovir

Question 197

A 56-year-old man is admitted with massive painless haematemesis. He gives a twenty-year history of alcohol abuse. He is jaundiced with multiple spider naevi, hypotensive, confused and has demonstrable shifting dullness. Which two of the following are true?

A a subclavian line should be inserted as soon as possible

B the patient should be commenced immediately on chlordiazepoxide or chlormethiazole to cover alcohol withdrawal

C thrombocytopaenia is highly suggestive of portal hypertension.

D urgent therapeutic paracentesis should be considered

E bacterial sensitivities on blood and ascitic cultures should be awaited before commencing antibiotics

F there is no role for medical therapies

G transjugular intrahepatic portosystemic stent-shunt (TIPSS) should only be considered if the patient is a transplant candidate

H statistically, in this patient, peptic ulcer disease is more likely than varices

I if oesophageal varices are present, injection sclerotherapy is the intervention of choice

J unless contraindicated, the patient should be treated with a beta-blocker after they have recovered from this episode

Question 198

As part of a routine health check, a young woman is found to have the following liver function tests: Bilirubin 37 µmol/L (normal range, 0–18), AST 14 IU/L (5–40), ALT 26 IU/L (5–45), alkaline phosphatase 125 IU/L, Albumin 40 g/L (36–45). Her haemoglobin is 13.7 g/dL (11.5–15.5) and reticulocyte count 1.2%. What is the most likely diagnosis?

A chronic alcoholic liver disease

B autoimmune haemolytic anaemia

C common bile duct stone

D Gilbert's syndrome

E primary biliary cirrhosis

Question 199

A 23-year-old woman is referred to clinic because her GP thinks she has developed acute hepatitis B. Which of the following investigations done when she became jaundiced is consistent with this diagnosis?

A HB core antibody positive and surface antibody positive

B HbsAb positive and core antibody negative

C HbsAg and HBeAg positive

D an alkaline phosphatase of 800 IU/L and an ALT of 50 IU/L

E HBsAg positive and e antibody positive

Question 200

An 84-year-old woman presents to the Accident and Emergency department with confusion and epigastric discomfort. She is not hypoxic. Liver function tests are abnormal: bilirubin 120 µmol/l, alkaline phosphatase 750 IU/L and AST 110 IU/L. Her CRP is raised at 120 mg/l. An ultrasound shows gallstones in the gallbladder and a mildly dilated common bile duct but no intraduct stones. The most likely diagnosis is:

A carcinoma of pancreas

B cholecystitis

C cholangitis

D ampullary carcinoma

E primary sclerosing cholangitis

Question 201

A 32-year-old woman is referred to the gastroenterology clinic with lethargy and mild elevation of her serum alanine aminotransferase (ALT 85 IU/L; normal < 40). Other investigations include aspartate aminotransferase 80 IU/L, GGT 60 IU/L (normal < 40). The bilirubin, alkaline phosphatase, albumin and prothrombin time are normal. Her full blood count is normal and the MCV is 85 fL. What is the most likely diagnosis?

A chronic hepatitis C

B alcoholic hepatitis

C primary biliary cirrhosis

D haemochromatosis

E Wilson's disease

Question 202

A 45-year-old man with a past history of chronic alcohol abuse is brought to the Accident and Emergency department after vomiting one litre of fresh red blood. Blood pressure on arrival is 90/40 mmHg with pulse 110/min. He is jaundiced and has multiple spider naevi and ascites. Which of the following drugs is most likely to be beneficial in his initial treatment?

A intravenous ranitidine

B oral propranolol

C intravenous terlipressin

D intravenous proton pump inhibitor

E helicobacter eradication therapy

Question 203

A 43-year-old woman with a long history of non-insulin dependent diabetes mellitus is noted to have an alanine aminotransferase (ALT) that is twice the upper limit of normal on routine screening. She says that she does not drink alcohol and never has done. She is obese (BMI 28). Which of the following is the most likely cause for her elevated ALT?

A haemochromatosis

B gall stones

C alcohol consumption

D hepatic steatosis

E drug-induced hepatitis

Question 204

In a patient who is jaundiced and HBsAg and HBeAg positive with evidence of cirrhosis (ascites) and an albumin of 28 g/L and a prothrombin time of 21 sec, the best treatment would be:

A ribavirin and alpha-interferon

B ribavirin

C lamivudine

D beta-interferon

E alpha-interferon

Question 205

A 50-year-old man with alcoholic cirrhosis is admitted with diuretic resistant ascites. Initial investigations show Na 127 mmol/l, creatinine 90 μmol/l, bilirubin 110 μmol/l, prothrombin time 18 seconds, albumin 27g/l. Which one of the following drugs should be avoided?

A flucloxacillin

B non-steroidal anti-inflammatory drugs (NSAIDs)

C paracetamol

D rifampicin

E chlordiazepoxide

Question 206

A 76-year-old man with a long history of rheumatoid arthritis is admitted after a haematemesis. His full blood count is as follows: Hb 10.8 g/dl, MCV 86 fl, WBC 7.4, platelets 243. Which of the following statements is true?

A The normal platelet count makes it unlikely that he has had a significant gastrointestinal bleed

B The normal blood count is reassuring: he is unlikely to have had a significant gastrointestinal bleed

C The blood count does not tell you whether or not he has had a significant gastrointestinal bleed

D The blood count suggests iron deficiency anaemia

E The high platelet count is consistent with recent gastrointestinal haemorrhage, but could also reflect activity of his arthritis

Question 207

A 54-year-old man is admitted following a haematemesis. You telephone the gastroenterologist on call to request an urgent endoscopy. He asks you what the patient's Rockall Score is. This is calculated on the basis of:

A co-morbidity, age, peripheral perfusion, systolic BP

B co-morbidity, age, pulse, systolic BP

C age, pulse, mean BP

D co-morbidity, age, peripheral perfusion, pulse, systolic BP

E previous history GI bleed, age, pulse, mean BP

Question 208

Upper gastrointestinal endoscopy reveals antral gastritis in a patient with duodenal ulceration, but a urease test for *Helicobacter pylori* is negative. The patient should be:

A investigated for other causes of duodenal ulceration with a fasting gastrin level

B managed with a proton pump inhibitor (PPI) alone

C treated with eradication therapy nevertheless

D offered surgery as a definitive cure

E given a repeat endoscopy in 3 months

Neurology

Gillian L Hall, Aroon D Hingorani,
John P Patten, Sivakumar Sathasivam
and Nick Ward *(Editor)*

Neurology

Answers are on pp. 154–155.

Question 209

A 38-year-old woman presents with sudden onset of diplopia. Figure 27 shows the appearance of her eyes. What is the diagnosis?

A right third nerve palsy

B right fourth nerve palsy

C right sixth nerve palsy

D internuclear ophthalmoplegia

E left medial rectus palsy

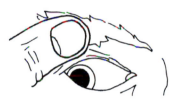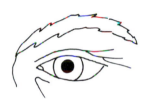

Fig. 27 Question 209.

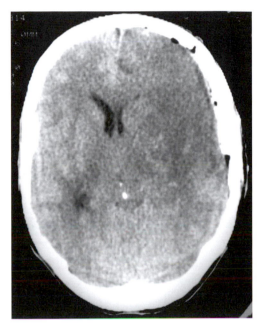

Fig. 28 Question 210.

Question 210

A 68-year-old man is found unresponsive by his wife in bed in the morning. An ambulance is called, and you are asked to assess him when he arrives in the Accident and Emergency department. His GCS is 7/15 and he makes no movement at all of his right arm or right leg. An urgent CT scan is done (see Figure 28). What is the diagnosis?

A subarachnoid haemorrhage

B cerebral oedema

C left middle cerebral artery infarction

D intracerebral haemorrhage

E right middle cerebral artery infarction

Question 211

A 60-year-old man is found to have a parietal lobe tumour. Which two of the following would you expect to find in this patient?

A ataxia

B bitemporal hemianopia

C contralateral motor weakness

D contralateral sensory disturbance

E dysphasia

F memory disturbance

G contralateral neglect

H nystagmus

I personality change

J spastic paraparesis

Question 212

You are asked to see a 36-year-old woman with headaches. Which two of the following features would suggest a diagnosis of tension-type headache?

A aggravated by physical activity

B associated with ptosis

C attacks commonly occur at a frequency of 20–40 times a day

D aura prior to headache

E bifronto-temporal pain

F commonly associated with vomiting

G headache relieved by alcohol

H lancinating pain

I regular aspirin is beneficial for pain relief

J throbbing pulsatile pain

Question 213

A 43-year-old man is referred after an episode of limb paralysis occurring suddenly at night-time. He describes waking shortly after falling asleep and being unable to move his limbs or to shout out for help. In addition he describes feeling as if he could not breathe properly. Symptoms lasted for about a minute. His father recently died from a stroke during sleep. He has no other symptoms apart from daytime sleepiness, which he puts down to working long hours. Blood pressure is 140/90 mmHg. There are no other abnormalities on examination. What is the most likely diagnosis?

A cervical disc prolapse

B depression and anxiety

C brainstem transient ischaemic attack

D nocturnal seizures

E narcolepsy

Question 214

A 70-year-old man presents with left-sided hemiparesis associated with a gaze paralysis to the right. Which part of the brain is damaged?

A left frontal lobe

B left pons

C right frontal lobe

D right medulla oblongata

E right pons

Question 215

A 67-year-old man attends the Accident and Emergency department after experiencing sudden onset left-sided weakness lasting for 20 minutes. Three days previously he had suffered an episode of blurred vision in his right eye that lasted for 5 minutes and was associated with a headache lasting for an hour. Previously he had been seeing his general practitioner for elevated blood pressure and for help in stopping smoking. Neurological examination is normal. His blood pressure is 150/90 mmHg, heart rate 84/min and regular. There are no carotid bruits. Which of the following is the most likely diagnosis?

A transient ischaemic attack secondary to giant cell arteritis

B migraine equivalent

C transient ischaemic attack secondary to carotid artery disease

D transient ischaemic attack secondary to small vessel disease

E transient ischaemic attack secondary to cardioembolism.

Question 216

The daughter of a 62-year-old man takes him to the Accident and Emergency department where you are asked to see him. Early that morning he developed a clumsy right hand and difficulty speaking, the problem with his hand having now persisted for 12 hours. He is known to have hypertension, asthma and rheumatoid arthritis. In addition he suffered from migraines as a young man. He smokes a pipe. On examination he has some weakness of the intrinsic muscles of the right hand. Visual fields, speech and sensation are normal. Blood pressure is 190/90 mmHg. Which of the following is the most likely diagnosis?

A left hemisphere lacunar stroke

B migraine equivalent

C left middle cerebral artery territory cardioembolic stroke

D left pontine microhaemorrhage

E neck-tongue syndrome

Question 217

A 46-year-old man presents with a headache over the left eye spreading across the forehead. It started suddenly and built up over three hours. He smokes 25 cigarettes a day. On examination he has a mild left ptosis and a small reactive left pupil. There are no other abnormal signs. What is the most likely diagnosis?

A basilar artery aneurysm

B internal carotid artery dissection

C migraine

D subarachnoid haemorrhage

E vertebral artery dissection

Question 218

A 37-year-old man is admitted one hour after the sudden onset of severe headache, which he described as like 'being hit on the head with a hammer'. You suspect subarachnoid haemorrhage, but a CT scan of the brain is reported as normal. To pursue the diagnosis you should:

A wait for 24 hours after the onset of headache, then perform a lumbar puncture to look for xanthochromia

B repeat the CT scan

C perform a lumbar puncture to look for xanthochromia as soon as possible

D perform a lumbar puncture to look for red blood cells in the CSF as soon as possible

E refer to neuroradiologist for cerebral angiography.

Question 219

A 70-year-old man is referred for increasing forgetfulness. On closer questioning, he admits to some urinary incontinence and unsteadiness on walking. He smokes 40 cigarettes a day and has been a heavy drinker in the past. What is most likely diagnosis?

A alcoholic cerebellar degeneration

B Alzheimer's disease

C frontotemporal dementia

D multi-infarct dementia

E normal pressure hydrocephalus

Question 220

An 84-year-old man presents with a 6-month history of increasing confusion, visual hallucinations, reduced mobility and falls. Which type of dementia fits this history best?

A Alzheimer's disease

B Pick's disease

C dementia with Lewy bodies

D Parkinson's disease

E vascular dementia

Question 221

A 60-year-old man is referred with stiffness and fluctuating confusion. His symptoms began about three years ago when he noticed stiffness in his legs which gradually progressed to affect all limbs. He now has a mild tremor affecting arms and legs, his writing has become illegible, and over the last six months he has developed hallucinations and reports seeing insects on the walls of his house. He is increasingly forgetful and his wife says that he is often restless and agitated at night. On examination his mini-mental test score is 15/30. Blood pressure fluctuates between 140–160/80–100 mmHg with no consistent postural drop. He is symmetrically rigid and slow with a tremor in all limbs. Cranial nerve examination reveals mild restriction of conjugate upgaze eye movement. His gait is shuffling with a tendency to fall backwards. What is the most likely diagnosis?

A benign essential tremor

B idiopathic Parkinson's disease

C Lewy body dementia

D multiple system atrophy

E progressive supranuclear palsy

Question 222

A recently married 26-year-old woman presents with a 2-month history of recurrent episodes of a rising epigastric sensation followed by lip-smacking and chewing movements with loss of awareness. The most likely diagnosis and the most appropriate investigation are:

A frontal lobe epilepsy and EEG

B migraine and anti-cardiolipin antibodies

C transient ischaemic attacks and CT scan

D multiple sclerosis and MRI brain scan

E temporal lobe epilepsy and MRI brain scan

Ophthalmology

Peggy Frith *(Editor)* and Hamish MA Towler

Ophthalmology

Answers are on pp. 155–156.

Question 223

A 45-year-old woman presents with blurred vision in her left eye. She has type 2 diabetes mellitus and a history of breast cancer treated by surgery and local radiotherapy 3 years previously. Her regular medications are gliclazide, tamoxifen and aspirin. Her blood pressure is 160/100 mmHg. Visual acuity in the left eye is 6/12 and the image (Figure 29) shows the optic fundus. What is the diagnosis?

A choroidal metastases
B tamoxifen retinopathy
C background diabetic retinopathy
D proliferative diabetic retinopathy
E hypertensive retinopathy

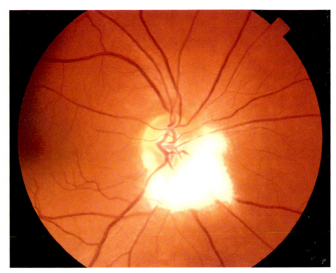

Fig. 30 Question 224.

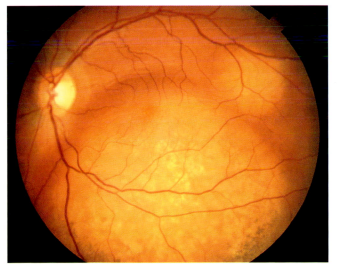

Fig. 29 Question 223.

Question 224

A 38-year-old man presents with a 5 day history of fever and headache. He is febrile (37.8°C) and hypertensive (blood pressure 170/105 mmHg), but examination is otherwise unremarkable excepting for a soft systolic murmur heard in the aortic area and an unusual appearance of his right optic fundus (see Figure 30). What is the cause of the fundal appearance?

A papilloedema
B toxoplasma chorioretinitis
C a Roth spot
D myelinated nerve fibres
E optic atrophy

Question 225

A 28-year-old woman with a ten year history of type 1 diabetes mellitus has the following fundal photograph (see Figure 31) taken at a routine eye check. Which of the following statements is correct?

A there is proliferative retinopathy, pre-retinal haemorrhage, macula oedema and scars of laser photocoagulation
B there is proliferative retinopathy, pre-retinal haemorrhage and scars of laser photocoagulation
C there is background retinopathy, pre-retinal haemorrhage and scars of laser photocoagulation
D there is proliferative retinopathy, pre-retinal haemorrhage and macula oedema
E there is background retinopathy, pre-retinal haemorrhage, macula oedema and scars of laser photocoagulation

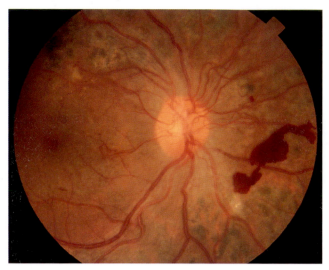

Fig. 31 Question 225.

Question 226

A middle-aged Afro-Caribbean woman presents with a history of fatigue, widespread joint pains and shortness of breath with a dry cough. Her ears and sinuses have been normal, but she mentions that she has recently attended the local eye casualty department with a painful, photophobic red eye. This was successfully treated with dexamethasone (Maxidex) drops hourly during the day, and another drop to dilate the pupil at night. The most convincing diagnostic possibility is:

A rheumatoid arthritis

B sarcoidosis

C Wegener's granulomatosis

D relapsing polychondritis

E ankylosing spondylitis

Question 227

A 60-year-old diabetic woman complains that her reading vision has become distorted in one eye and the image appears smaller than with the other eye. She has been diabetic for fifteen years and has maintained quite good diabetic control on diet and oral medication, with normal weight, blood pressure and plasma lipids. She is a non-smoker. What is the diagnosis?

A proliferative diabetic retinopathy

B diabetic maculopathy

C cataract

D retinal vein occlusion

E complication of oral hypoglycaemic medication.

Question 228

A middle-aged man reports that his vision has gradually become blurred, especially in the right eye. He is finding it difficult to read, even in bright light, and has great difficulty when driving at night because of glare from oncoming headlights. He had a successful renal transplant seven years ago and is on low dose maintenance immunosuppression and antihypertensive medication. His mother had renal failure and glaucoma. What is the diagnosis?

A iritis

B retinitis pigmentosa, related to the underlying cause of renal failure

C glaucoma

D cataract

E side effect of antihypertensive medication

Psychiatry

Vincent Kirchner and
Maurice Lipsedge *(Editor)*

Psychiatry

Answers are on pp. 156–157.

Question 229

A 46-year-old woman with pancreatic cancer attends clinic. Her pain is now well controlled on methadone, but she spends much of the day in bed and is refusing food. What are the two most helpful factors in distinguishing depression from the disease process and appropriate sadness?

A anorexia

B weight loss

C hypersomnia

D social withdrawal

E feelings of worthlessness

F nocturnal wakening

G fatigue

H anhedonia

I reduction in normal activities

J thoughts of death

Question 230

A 30-year-old man is involved in a multiple car crash in which several people die. He is not physically injured himself, but in the days that immediately follow he feels numb and detached, dazed and disorientated, with physical symptoms of sweating and shakiness. The most likely diagnosis is:

A acute stress disorder

B post-traumatic stress disorder

C adjustment disorder

D panic attack

E depression

Question 231

A 34-year-old woman develops chest pain after an argument with her 17-year-old daughter. She is brought to the Accident and Emergency department where you are asked to see her. She is hyperventilating and looks very anxious. She is tender to light pressure on the front of her chest, but examination is otherwise unremarkable. Breathing room air, her oxygen saturation (finger probe) is 99%. Her ECG is normal. You should:

A check troponin, plan to repeat ECG in 2 hours, and explain that you think that there is probably nothing serious going on, but you want to make sure that she has not had a heart attack

B check D-dimer and troponin, explain that you think that there is probably nothing serious going on, but you want to make sure that she has not had a clot of blood in the lung or a heart attack

C explain to her that she may be having a heart attack and that you wish to admit her to the coronary care unit for close monitoring

D explain to her that you are going to ask one of the nurses to put a paper bag over her head to help her breathing

E explain that she has had a panic attack and that her symptoms are a consequence of this, help her to control her breathing rate, and say that you think everything will settle down and she will be able to go home

Question 232

A 28-year-old woman is brought to the Accident and Emergency department after taking an overdose of 12×10 mg temazepam tablets. In assessing her risk of suicide, which of the following statements is FALSE?

A if she seems to have memory impairment, then her risk of suicide is relatively high

B the overdose is not life-threatening, indicating that her risk of suicide is relatively low

C if she had prepared by hoarding tablets, then her risk of suicide is relatively high

D if she has insomnia, then her risk of suicide is relatively high

E a past history of deliberate self harm (DSH) means that she has a relatively high risk of suicide

Question 233

A 34-year-old woman is brought into the Accident and Emergency department after taking an uncertain quantity of paracetamol two hours previously and trying to hang herself. She becomes agitated and insists that she wants to go home immediately. You judge that she is at high risk of suicide. How should you proceed?

A call the duty psychiatrist, and with other staff in the Accident and Emergency department attempt to restrain her under English Common Law until he or she arrives

B ask her to sign a 'discharge against medical advice' form and let her go

C call the duty psychiatrist, but let the patient go if she insists and the duty psychiatrist does not arrive in time to see her

D detain her under section 5(2) of the Mental Health Act

E call the hospital security services, restrain her and sedate her

Question 234

You are asked to see a 52-year-old woman with metastatic breast cancer who is tearful and feels that she can no longer cope. What would be the most appropriate course of action?

A screen for depression/suicidal thoughts and liaise with primary care team

B prescribe antidepressants

C reassure her that these feelings are normal in this situation

D listen to her concerns and refer her for counselling

E refer her for psychiatric assessment

Endocrinology

Anna Crown, Paul D Flynn,
Mark Gurnell *(Editor)* and
Mohammed Z Qureshi

Endocrinology

Answers are on pp. 157–160.

Question 235

A 17-year-old young woman has never had any menstrual periods. She is generally fit and well, but says that she does not like cold weather and admits to being a 'faddy eater'. She is short (5 ft 2 ins, 157 cm tall), as are her parents. Her image is shown in Figure 32. What is the most likely diagnosis?

A hypothyroidism
B constitutional short stature
C anorexia nervosa
D Turner's syndrome
E coeliac disease

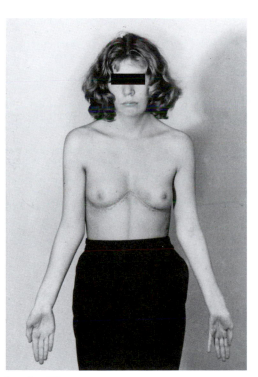

Fig. 32 Question 235.

Question 236

A 48-year-old woman with a history of asthma treated with regular inhaled steroid and inhaled salbutamol as needed, and with occasional use of oral prednisolone at the time of acute exacerbation, is referred as an outpatient with weight gain and new onset of diabetes. Her face is shown in Figure 33. The most appropriate course of action would be:

A stop oral and inhaled steroid and arrange to review in 3 months
B perform 24 hour urinary free cortisol estimation
C estimate plasma ACTH level
D arrange CT brain
E perform short synacthen test

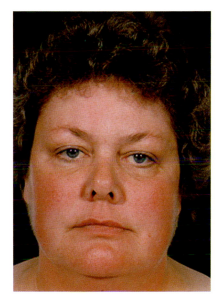

Fig. 33 Question 236.

Question 237

A 45-year-old taxi driver is seen in the outpatient clinic with recently diagnosed moderate to severe hypertension. He has no significant past medical history and says that he is not taking any medications. His serum potassium levels have been persistently low (2.5–3.2 mmol/l), his plasma renin activity (PRA) is suppressed and a concomitant aldosterone level is significantly raised. Which two of the following conditions are most likely to be present?

A phaeochromocytoma
B renal artery stenosis
C coarctation of aorta

D idiopathic hyperaldosteronism (bilateral adrenal zona glomerulosa hyperplasia)

E essential hypertension

F diuretic treatment (concealed)

G carcinoid syndrome

H Conn's syndrome

I excessive liquorice ingestion

J Cushing's syndrome

Question 238

A 31-year-old, 76 kg, type 1 diabetic man is admitted as a medical emergency with a 24-hour history of central abdominal pain, nausea and vomiting. Plasma glucose is 29.3 mmol/l and other routine blood tests show Haemoglobin 16.1 g/dl, WBC 19.3 × 10^9/l, plts 380 × 10^9/l, Na 127 mmol/l, K 6.4 mmol/l, Urea 15.2 mmol/l, creatinine 124 µmol/l, amylase 380 iu/l (normal < 50), urine ketostix reaction +++. Arterial blood gas analysis reveals pH 7.1, pCO$_2$ 2.8 kPa, pO$_2$ 25.1 kPa, HCO$_3$- 12 mmol/l, base excess –16. Choose the two correct statements from the following list:

A the raised white blood cell count makes infection the most likely precipitant of diabetic ketoacidosis (DKA) in this case

B the amylase suggests pancreatitis as the likely precipitant of DKA in this case

C his fluid deficit is likely to be around 7 L

D bicarbonate therapy is indicated

E whole body potassium levels are increased

F phosphate concentrations are likely to be increased because of renal impairment

G the principal role of insulin therapy is to increase glucose uptake into peripheral tissues and liver

H the principal role of insulin therapy is to inhibit lipolysis and gluconeogenesis

I the low sodium concentration is entirely due to renal losses

J the principal ketone body in plasma and urine in DKA is acetoacetate

Question 239

A 55-year-old man with type 2 diabetes who smokes 10–15 cigarettes/day is referred to the joint diabetic/renal clinic by his general practitioner who has documented proteinuria of 1.5 gm/24 hours and a serum creatinine of 255 µmol/l. He takes three antihypertensive agents and his blood pressure is averaging 140/80 mmHg. His cholesterol is 6.4 mmol/l and high-density lipoprotein

(HDL) 0.9 mmol/l. His anti-diabetic therapy includes metformin and gliclazide and his last HbA1c was 6.7%. Which two of the following steps are most appropriate at this clinic visit?

A commence insulin therapy

B refer for renal dialysis

C arrange for renal biopsy

D anticoagulate with warfarin

E start a statin (HMG Co-A reductase inhibitor)

F stop metformin

G increase antihypertensive medication

H commence a low protein diet

I stop gliclazide

J start diuretic therapy

Question 240

A 27-year-old woman is referred with hirsutism. Which one of the following features from her history would be of most concern?

A history of hirsutism dating back six months

B family history of hirsutism

C family history of infertility

D the use of oral corticosteroids to control asthma

E weight gain over preceding six months

Question 241

A 58-year-old woman has mild hypertension (150/95 mmHg) and hypokalaemia (serum potassium 3.1 mmol/l). She is found to have bilateral adrenal hyperplasia. What is the most appropriate treatment?

A oral potassium supplements

B bilateral adrenalectomy

C spironolactone

D carbenoxolone

E glucocorticoids

Question 242

A 31-year-old man is referred to the endocrinology clinic for investigation of infertility with azoospermia. He has no other complaints and looks well and suntanned. His LH and FSH are suppressed, and his testosterone is 28 nmol/l (normal 10–40 nmol/l). Which one of the following investigations would be most appropriate to do next?

A pituitary MRI

B midnight 17 hydroxyprogesterone

C karyotype

D transferrin saturation

E testicular ultrasonography

Question 243

A 40-year-old medical secretary is being investigated for hypertension. Her 24-hour urinary free cortisol levels are high on two occasions and she has significantly raised serum cortisol levels with loss of diurnal rhythm. Which one of the following features would favour benign adrenal adenoma as the cause of her Cushing's syndrome over other possible causes?

A presence of hypokalaemia

B absence of hirsutism

C presence of weight loss

D absence of typical features of Cushing's syndrome

E normal MRI of the pituitary gland

Question 244

A 54-year-old man is followed up in the endocrine clinic following bilateral adrenalectomy 25 years previously for Cushing's disease. He is on hydrocortisone 20 mg in the morning and 10 mg at teatime, and 200 micrograms of fludrocortisone a day. His most recent cortisol day profile is satisfactory. His serum sodium is 149 mmol/l and potassium 3.2 mmol/l. His blood pressure, on two occasions, is greater than 170/100 mmHg. What action will you take?

A reduce hydrocortisone dose to half

B start antihypertensive treatment

C reduce fludrocortisone to 100 micrograms a day

D start at a small dose of spironolactone and gradually increase

E advise a low salt diet and review in clinic

Question 245

A 44-year-old woman with hypertension is referred as an outpatient. You suspect she may have primary hyperaldosteronism. Which one of the following would point AWAY from this diagnosis?

A a low plasma renin level

B hypokalaemia

C polyuria

D acidosis

E a good response to spironolactone

Question 246

A 62-year-old man is found to have glycosuria on a routine urine test. His blood glucose is 21 mmol/l and a diagnosis of maturity onset diabetes mellitus is made. He is very concerned about the implications for his United Kingdom driving licence: which one of the following statements is true?

A tablet-treated diabetic patients are allowed up to a 3-year licence

B insulin-treated diabetic patients are allowed up to a 3-year licence

C diet-controlled diabetic patients are allowed up to a 5-year licence

D insulin-treated gestational diabetes patients are not allowed to drive

E diabetic patients with eyesight complications have separate rules to non-diabetic patients

Question 247

A 55-year-old man with type 2 diabetes mellitus, who has been lost to follow-up for over 2 years, is admitted with poorly controlled diabetes. Apart from polyuria, polydipsia and tiredness, he also complains of blurred vision, especially in right eye. He has lost weight but has dependent oedema of his lower legs. His urine dipstix test reveals 4+ proteinuria and 4+ glycosuria. He has signs of peripheral neuropathy and a right Charcot's foot. His laboratory results are as follows: haemoglobin 11 g/dl, MCV 84, WBC 9.0×10^9/l, platelets 323×10^9/l, ESR 18 mm/hour, sodium 138 mmol/l, potassium 4.7 mmol/l, urea 11.8 mmol/l, creatinine 198 µmol/l, albumin 32 g/l, HbA1c 11.9%. Which one of the following actions / tests should be your highest priority?

A urinary albumin:creatinine ratio

B radiograph right foot

C fundoscopy through dilated pupils

D ultrasound scan of renal tract

E 24-hour urinary protein estimation

Question 248

A 62-year-old man with type 2 diabetes for 17 years is found to have decreased visual acuity at annual review. Which one of the following statements about maculopathy is true?

A maculopathy causes loss of peripheral vision

B maculopathy requires routine referral for an ophthalmology opinion

C maculopathy is unaffected by poor glycaemic control

D circinate exudates may indicate maculopathy

E maculopathy is unaffected by hypertension

Question 249

A 72-year-old woman is admitted with headaches, polyuria and polydipsia of recent onset. She has previously had a mastectomy for breast cancer. A CT head scan shows multiple cerebral metastases. Admission laboratory results reveal sodium 153 mmol/l, potassium 4.0 mmol/l, urea 5.0 mmol/l, creatinine 110 µmol/l and glucose 5 mmol/l. Her 24 hour urinary volume is 4.4 litres with plasma osmolality 320 mOsm/kg and urinary osmolality 254 mOsm/kg. Which one of the following treatments will you use?

A hypotonic saline
B hydrochlorothiazide
C desmopressin (DDAVP)
D demeclocycline
E water restriction

Nephrology

Nick C Fluck, Philip Kalra, Patrick H Maxwell
(Editor) **and Chris A O'Callaghan**

Nephrology

Answers are on pp. 160–162.

Question 250

A 68-year-old man undergoes emergency repair of a ruptured abdominal aortic aneurysm. After surgery he is transferred to the intensive care unit for ventilation. Over the next 24 hours he passes very little urine. Figure 34 shows one of his feet. Which one of the following conditions that affect the kidney is suggested by this appearance of his foot?

A acute tubular necrosis

B acute cortical necrosis

C vasculitis

D rapidly progressive glomerulonephritis

E cholesterol embolisation

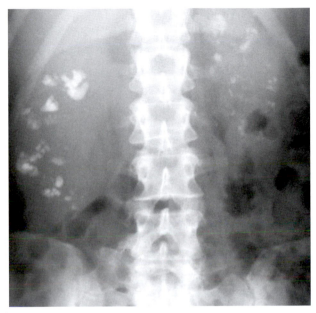

Fig. 35 Question 251.

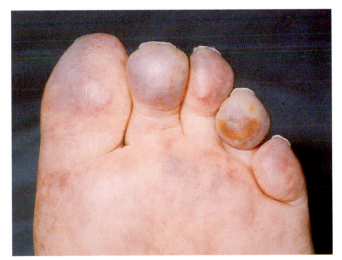

Fig. 34 Question 250.

Question 251

A 48-year-old man with no significant past medical history but who takes occasional doses of antacid for indigestion presents following an episode of right-sided renal colic, following which he passed a small urinary stone. His abdominal radiograph is shown (see Figure 35). What is the likely diagnosis?

A medullary sponge kidney

B cystinuria

C urate nephropathy

D milk-alkali syndrome

E cortical necrosis

Question 252

A 47-year-old woman presents with oedema. She has a 20-year history of rheumatoid arthritis causing severe joint destruction. Her 24-hour urinary protein excretion is 6 grams and her serum creatinine is 565 µmol/l. Which two of the following are the most likely diagnoses?

A polycystic kidney disease

B AL amyloidosis

C cystinuria

D AA amyloidosis

E haemolytic uraemic syndrome

F membranous nephropathy

G renal artery stenosis

H Takayasu's disease

I medullary sponge kidney

J focal segmental proliferative glomerulonephritis

113

Question 253

A 73-year-old woman presents with a 6-month history of malaise, anorexia, progressive leg swelling and easy bruising. Plasma creatinine is 97 µmol/l. 24 hour urinary protein excretion is 12 grams. Renal ultrasound shows two echogenic kidneys, both 10 cm in length. CRP is 5 mg/l (normal range <5). She has a 7 g/l IgG lambda paraprotein on serum electrophoresis, but no Bence Jones protein in the urine. Which two further investigations would be most appropriate?

A CT scan chest
B CT scan abdomen
C renal biopsy
D renal angiogram
E renal venogram
F bone marrow aspirate and trephine
G a serum amyloid P (SAP) scan
H isotope renography
I skin biopsy
J rectal biopsy

Question 254

A 40-year-old woman who has attended a well-woman clinic is found to have serum calcium 2.85 mmol/l and phosphate 0.65 mmol/l. Further investigations show that her intact parathyroid hormone (PTH) level is 9.0 pmol/l (normal range 1.1 to 6.8), and the 24-hour urinary calcium excretion is 0.9 mmol/l (normal range 2.5–7.5). Plasma creatinine and alkaline phosphatase are both in the normal range. She says she thinks her father was found to have a high calcium level. Which of the following statements is correct?

A she should be screened for a mutation in the multiple endocrine neoplasia-1 (MEN-1) gene
B the most likely diagnosis is primary hyperparathyroidism
C parathyroid surgery is not indicated now but will be necessary in the future
D she probably has an abnormality of the calcium-sensing receptor
E treatment with oral phosphate supplements should suppress her PTH level

Question 255

In a patient with hypertension, which one of the following features is consistent with a clinical diagnosis of Liddle's syndrome (a mutation affecting the sodium channels in the distal tubules)?

A raised catecholamine levels
B high aldosterone levels
C skin nodules
D high renin levels
E hypokalaemia

Question 256

A 36-year-old man presents with microscopic haematuria and hypertension. Ultrasound scan shows several cysts in the kidneys, and two solid lesions, the larger of which is 5 cm diameter. The man is not in contact with his family, but he knows that his father died undergoing surgery for a brain tumour at the age of 30, also that one of his father's two sisters had some kind of kidney problem and was deaf in one ear. What is the most likely diagnosis?

A Alport's syndrome
B adult polycystic kidney disease
C tuberous sclerosis
D von Hippel Lindau disease
E Fabry's disease

Question 257

An anxious 52-year-old woman has adult polycystic kidney disease. She shows you a long list of things that she says are associated with this condition. Which of the following is NOT a recognised association?

A subarachnoid haemorrhage
B cerebellar cysts
C liver cysts
D colonic diverticuli
E mitral valve prolapse

Question 258

A 31-year-old woman presents with leg oedema that extends to her groins. Urine dipstick analysis shows proteinuria 4 +. Blood tests reveal normal renal excretory function (creatinine 68 µmol/l) but severe hypoalbuminaemia (albumin 12 g/l). A renal biopsy is reported as normal other than showing foot process fusion on electron microscopy. Which one of the following agents would NOT be appropriate as part of her initial therapy?

A ciclosporin
B furosemide
C simvastatin
D warfarin
E prednisolone

Question 259

A 30-year-old man with no antecedent illness presents with severely raised BP (150/110 mm Hg), frothy urine, peripheral oedema and lethargy. There is +++ blood and ++++ protein on urinalysis. 24-hour urinary protein loss is 6.6 grams. Plasma albumin is 28 g/L. Plasma C3 is 0.10 (low). Plasma creatinine is 145 µmol/l. Which of the following renal lesions is most likely to be found on renal biopsy?

A IgA nephropathy

B membranous glomerulonephritis

C focal segmental glomerulosclerosis

D post infectious glomerulonephritis

E mesangiocapillary glomerulonephritis

Question 260

A 23-year-old man presents with a rash on his legs. Stick testing of his urine reveals proteinuria + and haematuria +++. What is the most likely diagnosis?

A Henoch-Schönlein purpura

B mixed essential cryoglobulinaemia

C minimal change nephropathy

D IgA nephropathy

E membranous glomerulonephritis

Question 261

A 42-year-old woman presents with a plasma creatinine of 240 µmol/l and 3 g of proteinuria per 24 hours. She weighs 148 kg, hence a renal biopsy is not possible because of her size. What is the most likely diagnosis?

A minimal change nephropathy

B focal segmental glomerulosclerosis

C membranous nephropathy

D Bartter's syndrome

E myeloma

Question 262

A 53-year-old man presents having felt unwell for several weeks with general malaise and fatigue. He has had recurrent sinusitis for over a year and occasionally noticed a rash on his chest. Routine blood tests show that he has a serum creatinine of 180 µmol/l. Which of the following is the most likely diagnosis?

A chronic renal failure

B systemic vasculitis

C minimal change nephropathy

D urinary tract infection

E focal segmental glomerulosclerosis

Question 263

In a patient with diabetes mellitus and a serum creatinine of 210 µmol/l, which one of the following findings would lead you to suspect a diagnosis other than diabetic nephropathy?

A normal fundoscopy

B HbA1C of 8.1%

C normal-sized kidneys on ultrasound examination

D proteinuria of 1.2 g per 24 hours

E knowledge that the creatinine had been 110 µmol/l 18 months earlier

Question 264

A 23-year-old African woman presents with seizures, hypertension, a rash, a raised ESR, a normal CRP and a creatinine of 373 µmol/l. What is the most likely diagnosis?

A myeloma

B Hashimoto's disease

C systemic lupus erythematosus

D staphylococcal septicaemia

E sickle cell disease

Rheumatology and clinical immunology

Khalid Binymin, Hilary J Longhurst,
Siraj A Misbah *(Editor)* and
Neil Snowden

Rheumatology and Clinical Immunology

Answers are on pp. 162–164.

Question 265

The image (Figure 36) shows the hand of an 18-year-old man who presents to the Accident and Emergency department with a fever and a rash. What is the probable diagnosis?

A streptococcal septicaemia

B staphylococcal septicaemia

C meningococcal septicaemia

D thrombocytopenic purpura

E acute vasculitis

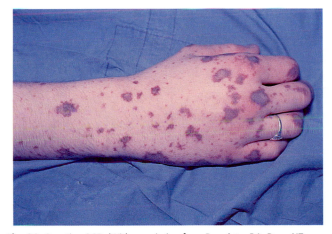

Fig. 36 Question 265. (With permission from Bannister BA, Begg NT, Gillespie SH. *Infectious Disease*, 2nd edn. Oxford: Blackwell Science, 2000.)

Question 266

A 30-year-old woman with a two-year history of Raynaud's phenomenon presents with increasing pain in her hand (Figure 37a). Her serum is tested for antinuclear antibodies on a human epithelial cell line (HEp-2) substrate, with result shown (Figure 37b). What is the likely diagnosis?

A Wegener's granulomatosis

B microscopic polyangiitis

C diffuse cutaneous systemic sclerosis

D limited cutaneous systemic sclerosis

E polyarteritis nodosa

Question 267

A 30-year-old garage mechanic presents with severe malaise that has come on over a week or so. He does not have any specific symptoms and examination is unremarkable, excepting that he looks unwell and is pale. Blood tests confirm that he is anaemic (Hb 8.7 g/dl), also that he is in renal failure (Na 135 mmol/l, K 5.8 mmol/l, creatinine 798 µmol/l). There is patchy lung shadowing on his chest radiograph. His kidneys are of normal size on ultrasound and renal biopsy is performed to achieve a diagnosis of the cause of his renal failure. The image (Figure 38) shows the appearance of the biopsy on immunofluorescent examination using an anti-IgG antibody. What is the diagnosis?

A Goodpasture's disease

B IgA nephropathy

C Wegener's granulomatosis

D membranous glomerulonephritis

E cholesterol embolisation

Question 268

A 58-year-old woman is referred with pain and stiffness in her hands and knees. She has a few patches of psoriasis on her arms. Her hands are shown in the picture (Figure 39). What are the two most likely diagnoses?

A gout

B nodal osteoarthritis

C pseudogout

D systemic sclerosis

E psoriatic arthritis

F systemic lupus erythematosus

G ankylosing spondylitis

H rheumatoid arthritis

I reactive arthritis

J SAPHO syndrome

Question 269

A 30-year-old woman presents with several attacks of pain and swelling affecting the metacarpophalangeal and proximal interphalangeal joints over the past few months, with morning stiffness and fatigue. What are the two most likely diagnoses?

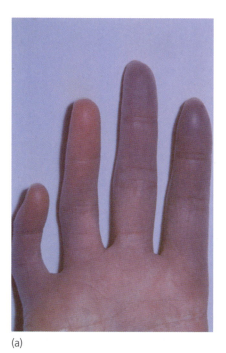

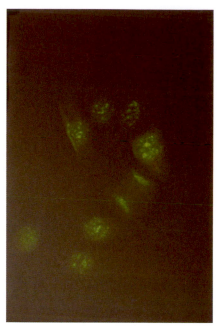

(a)   (b)   **Fig. 37** Question 266.

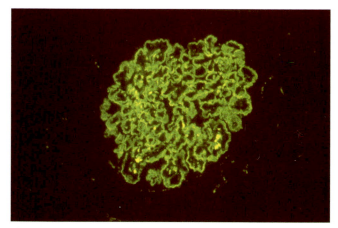

Fig. 38 Question 267.

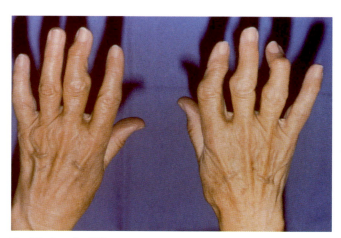

Fig. 39 Question 268.

A ankylosing spondylitis
B pseudogout
C systemic lupus erythematosus
D primary generalised osteoarthritis
E reactive arthritis
F gout
G rheumatoid arthritis
H psoriatic arthropathy
I systemic sclerosis
J rheumatic fever

Question 270

A 73-year-old man presents with a 24-hour history of a painful swollen left knee. He has had minor pain and stiffness in both knees for many years and now feels generally unwell. His temperature is 37.4°C. The most likely diagnosis is:

A gout
B pseudogout
C septic arthritis
D reactive arthritis
E rheumatoid arthritis

Question 271

A 60-year-old woman develops acute, severe low thoracic back pain. A radiograph shows a vertebral crush fracture. Which two of the following reduce an individual's risk for developing osteoporosis?

A early menarche
B early menopause
C smoking
D high alcohol intake
E prolonged treatment with corticosteroids
F rheumatoid arthritis
G Crohn's disease
H asthma
I frequent walks
J obesity

Question 272

A 48-year-old woman with a 10-year history of systemic sclerosis presents with exertional breathlessness. Serial peak flow rates are normal. A plain chest radiograph is reported as normal and pulmonary function tests reveal reduced gas transfer with a KCO 50% of predicted. Her haemoglobin is normal. She has never smoked. Which two of the following investigations are most likely to be helpful in determining the cause of her breathlessness?

A antinuclear antibody
B high resolution CT scan of the thorax
C antibodies to extractable nuclear antigens
D 24-hour blood pressure monitoring
E V/Q scanning
F serum lactate
G muscle biopsy
H barium swallow
I trial of corticosteroid treatment
J diaphragmatic function tests

Question 273

A 79-year-old man presents feeling very unwell with recent and sudden onset of severe pain and stiffness around his shoulders and hips. He was previously well and admits to no other symptoms, in particular no headache or visual disturbance. Examination shows painful, restricted shoulders and hips, but no myopathy. He has no lymph nodes or abdominal masses. Initial investigations show a normal blood count, biochemical profile, thyroid function, prostate specific antigen, MSU and chest radiograph. His ESR is 85 mm and CRP is 110 mg/l (normal < 10). Which two of the following statements give the best advice regarding his treatment? He should:

A be started on prednisolone 60 mg daily reduced over 12–18 months
B be treated with a Cox II inhibitor
C be started on prednisolone 15 mg daily for 2 weeks only
D be treated with alfacalcidol 2 µg daily
E be treated with low dose methotrexate
F be started on prednisolone 15 mg daily, tailed off over 12–18 months
G receive 3 × 1 g doses of i.v. methylprednisolone
H receive prophylactic treatment for osteoporosis
I receive simple analgesia
J receive prednisolone 60 mg daily for 1 month

Question 274

You are called to the Accident and Emergency department to review a 28-year-old woman with pleuritic chest pain. Which one of the following statements concerning this patient is true?

A low white cell count is consistent with systemic lupus erythematosus (SLE)
B low white cell count is not consistent with tuberculosis
C the presence of anticardiolipin antibodies IgG 17 GPLU/ml (NR < 14), IgM 21 MPLU/ml (NR < 10) suggests that she may have a pulmonary embolus
D the presence of antinuclear antibodies at a titre of 1/80 suggests that she may have a connective tissue disease
E the presence of antinuclear cytoplasmic antibodies (cANCA) at a titre of 1 in 20 suggests that Wegener's granulomatosis is likely

Question 275

A 20-year-old man presents with arthralgia, skin rash and haematuria. Renal biopsy shows focal necrotising glomerulonephritis with diffuse mesangial IgA deposits. What is the most likely diagnosis?

A systemic lupus erythematosus (SLE)
B Henoch–Schönlein purpura
C juvenile rheumatoid arthritis
D post-streptococcal glomerulonephritis
E Goodpasture's syndrome

Question 276

A 36-year-old woman is referred with a 1-year history of muscle pain, tiredness and sleep disturbance. She denies fever, weight loss and arthralgia. Examination reveals tenderness over her occiput, trapezius and lumbar area.

Her blood results show a normal ESR, CRP, FBC, a weakly positive ANA (1:80) and normal complement levels. What is the most likely diagnosis?

A polymyositis

B system lupus erythematous (SLE)

C Sjögren's syndrome

D polymyalgia rheumatica

E fibromyalgia

Question 277

A 30-year-old woman presents with a 6-month history of swelling and pain involving the distal interphalangeal joints of the hands. The ESR is 65 mm in the first hour. What is the most likely diagnosis?

A generalised osteoarthritis

B rheumatoid arthritis

C psoriatic arthritis

D systemic lupus erythematosus (SLE)

E gout

Question 278

A 68-year old man presents with sudden severe pain and swelling in the left knee. Synovial fluid analysis shows abundant calcium pyrophosphate dihydrate (CPPD) crystals. In his further assessment, which one of the following tests is NOT appropriate?

A creatinine kinase

B serum calcium

C thyroid function test

D serum ferritin level

E HbA$_1$C

Question 279

A 68-year-old woman with longstanding congestive cardiac failure (ejection fraction 20%) presents with a hot, swollen right knee. The following results are obtained: FBC normal, Urea 11 mM, Creatinine 196 μmol/l. Synovial fluid: many monosodium urate crystals seen on microscopy, culture sterile. What is the best treatment for her acute arthritis?

A allopurinol

B colchicine 0.5 mg every 2–4 hours

C indometacin 50 mg tds

D co-codamol 30/500 every 6 hours

E intra-articular corticosteroids

Question 280

A 70-year-old woman has a 17-year history of rheumatoid arthritis. She presents with recurrent attacks of red congested eyes with a sensation of grittiness. The most likely cause of her red eyes is likely to be:

A scleritis

B episcleritis

C keratitis

D keratoconjunctivitis sicca

E choroiditis

Question 281

A 77-year-old man presents with persistent headache and progressive deafness. On examination he has frontal bossing of the forehead and conductive deafness, more severe in the right ear. His serum alkaline phosphatase is significantly raised at 870 Iu/L. Which of the following statements is most accurate about this disease?

A it usually affects a single bone

B the skull is the most commonly affected bone

C bone pain is the most common presenting feature

D hearing loss is often due to involvement of the middle ear ossicles leading to conductive deafness

E bone pain is typically increased with rest and on weight bearing

Question 282

A 64-year-old man presents to the Accident and Emergency department with a 2-day history of increasing pain and swelling of his left knee. He denies a history of trauma. On examination, the knee is hot, red, swollen and extremely tender. Which of the following investigations is most important?

A plain radiograph of the knee

B blood cultures

C C-reactive protein (CRP)

D joint aspiration

E plasma uric acid level

Answers

Genetics and Molecular Medicine

Answer to Question 1

C

Imprinting is the term used to refer to the differential expression of alleles contingent on their parental origin.

The mechanism of imprinting is poorly understood, but it involves DNA methylation. Disease may occur as a result of a defect in only one allele if the other allele is imprinted and thus not expressed.

Some genetic disorders may be due to maternal imprinting (e.g. Prader-Willi syndrome) and some paternal (e.g. Angelman's syndrome).

Answer to Question 2

D

Recombination is the production of genetic combinations not found in either of the parents. In humans, this is predominantly created by crossing-over between homologous chromosomes during meiosis.

The maximum possible recombination distance between two genes (or any two markers on a chromosome) is 50%, because they may be inherited together at random on 50% of occasions. If two genes (or markers) have a recombination fraction of 50%, then they either lie on different chromosomes, or a long distance apart on the same chromosome.

Answer to Question 3

C

It is now possible to tell whether two bits of human DNA are linked (relatively close together on a chromosome) by reference to the map of the human genome. It was not possible to do this before the genome map was published, and the LOD score (LOD being an abbreviation for Logarithm of the Odds) was the most commonly used means of quantifying linkage. Based on analysis of data from pedigrees it provides a statistical measure of the chance that one bit of DNA (the putative gene for a disease trait in this instance) is linked to another (the known genetic locus).

Answer to Question 4

B

Translation is the name of the process of decoding protein sequence from messenger RNA (mRNA), the polypeptide amino acid sequence being determined by the base sequence of its mRNA. The RNA bases are 'read' in a 3 base pair or triplet code, each 3-base pair unit being referred to as a codon. The 'decoding' is performed by transfer RNA (tRNA) molecules, which recognise each codon by virtue of a complementary RNA sequence (the anticodon), which forms a unique part of each tRNA molecule.

Answer to Question 5

A

Between 20 and 30 base pairs upstream of the transcriptional start site (transcription being the process whereby a DNA sequence is converted into an RNA message) are promoter elements that bind RNA polymerases. The binding sequences for these polymerases are characteristic, with such a run of conserved sequences being called a 'consensus sequence'. One of the commonest of these sequences is a TATA box (consensus, TATAA).

Answer to Question 6

E

Single gene abnormalities may result in autosomal dominant and recessive disorders, or X-linked disorders. A Mendelian X-linked condition can affect, and be transmitted by, both males and females.

Affected females may be either heterozygous or homozygous for the mutant gene. If the disease is expressed in the female heterozygote it is referred to as X-linked dominant and if only in the female homozygote, then X-linked recessive. All males will express the full disease since they carry only one X chromosome. Affected females transmit the condition to half of their children, whether male or female. Affected males pass the defective X chromosome to all of their daughters, but to none of their sons (since no X chromosome is transmitted to them from their father). An X-linked dominant disorder should be observed in females twice as often as in males.

Answer to Question 7

D

PCR can only be used on a DNA template as the reaction employs a heat-stable DNA (Taq) polymerase. RNA can be amplified, but only after an initial reverse transcription reaction that generates copy DNA from the RNA. Taq polymerase and other related enzymes do make errors, but the frequency of these is known and not high enough to prevent PCR techniques being used diagnostically. Many genetic markers such as microsatellites and single nucleotide polymorphisms (SNPs) are amenable to PCR analysis, indeed it would be no understatement to say that PCR has revolutionised molecluar biology. The essence of PCR is geometric amplification and not linear amplification. For this reason, 30 cylces of PCR could theoretically amplify starting DNA by a factor of 2^{30}.

Answer to Question 8

E

Although human and other primates genomes are extremely close, primates are not commonly used in medical research. Experiments on primates can only be justified ethically and financially when work on less sentient organisms such as rodents, particularly mice, cannot provide an adequate model of human disease. In relation to humans, the organ system least well represented in the mouse is the central nervous system.

In studying genetic disease mice are also valuable because they can be subject to genetic manipulation. A transgenic mouse is one that carries inserted copies of a gene or sequence under investigation. The eradication or alteration of an existing gene locus can be carried out by generating a so called 'knock-out' in which a critical region of a gene sequence is altered in an embryonic stem cell and this altered stem cell is then re-introduced back into the embryo at the blastocyst stage.

Answer to Question 9

D

Linkage disequilibrium can be simply defined as the non-random association of alleles in a breeding population.

Linkage disequilibrium almost always, but not invariably, occurs between alleles at genetic loci that are closely linked in the genome. However, within any given population the extent and pattern linkage disequilibrium varies considerably depending on the time of origin of the alleles in question in that population, as well as the population history following on from the time at which the mutation arose.

The degree of linkage disequilibrium can be highly variable: in some cases the inheritance of one allele will exclude the inheritance of another neighbouring allele, but this is not necessarily the case.

Linkage disequilibrium depends entirely on the population history: it can exist between common and rare alleles, or vice versa. Some patterns of linkage disequilibrium will be shared between northern European and northern Indo-Asian populations, but the different 'experiences' that these populations have undergone since

they diverged are such that one cannot assume an extrapolation between one population and the other.

Answer to Question 10

B

The invariant pairing of nucleic acid bases in the DNA double helix first alerted Crick and Watson to the possibility that the DNA molecule in this form constituted the molecular basis of heredity. A purine always pairs with a pyrimidine (adenine with thymine; guanine with cytosine).

DNA is much more stable than RNA. This property is exploited in forensic pathology (and very fancifully in the plot line of Jurassic Park).

The bases in RNA and DNA differ. RNA contains uracil in place of thymidine; they are structurally similar. In RNA ribose is hydroxylated at the 2′ and 3′ positions; in DNA only at the 3′ position (hence 'deoxyribonucleic').

Paternal and maternal chromosomes contribute to the gene product in the vast majority of instances. However, this is not always the case; examples include the allelic exclusion seen in mature T and B lymphocytes, in which the majority of these cells express the antigen receptor from one allele only. Another example is seen in genomic regions, which are subject to 'imprinting'. In these areas only, genes from a defined parental origin are transcribed. Thus some imprinted genes are always from the maternal allele, others are invariably paternal.

Biochemistry and Metabolism

Answer to Question 11

A

Peptide bonds are linkages between the carboxylic acid group of one amino acid and the amino group of the next. These create the secondary structure of protein, which is the linear sequence of amino acids in the chain. The chain folds to create the tertiary structure of the protein that is critical for function. This tertiary structure is often stabilised by hydrogen bonds between amino acid side chains, but these do not constitute 'peptide bonds'.

Answer to Question 12

B

Glycogen is the storage form of carbohydrate, found predominantly in muscle and liver. Chains of glucose residues are linked by alpha-1,4 glycosidic bonds, i.e. between the first carbon of one glucose and the fourth carbon of the next. Branches occur about every ten residues, and are formed by alpha-1,6 glycosidic linkages.

Glycogen synthesis and degradation occur at the tips of branches, with the branching structure increasing the number of sites at which glucose residues can be added or removed.

Answer to Question 13

C

Fatty acids are built up from acetyl CoA units in the cytosol using energy derived from NADPH and ATP. The backbone is constructed on a carrier protein and is released when it is 16–18 carbons long.

The mechanism is as follows: acetyl CoA in the cytosol is carboxylated to malonyl CoA by an enzyme called acetyl CoA carboxylase, using energy derived from ATP and a carboxyl group from bicarbonate. This is the rate limiting step controlling the fatty acid synthetic pathway. The malonyl group is transferred from CoA to an acyl carrier protein, which then adds the two carbon malonyl unit to the growing acyl chain.

Answer to Question 14

D

Glycosaminoglycans are high molecular weight polysaccharides that are made up of chains of repeating disaccharide units, comprising an amino sugar (such as glucosamine or galactosamine) linked most commonly to a hexuronic acid (glucuronic acid or iduronic acid).

Glycosaminoglycans are usually linked together in a comb-like structure to a protein core, forming a proteoglycan.

Glycosaminoglycans are normally degraded in lysosomes. Inherited deficiencies of lysosomal enzymes can result in lysosomal storage diseases known as mucopolysaccharidoses, e.g. Hunter's and Hurler's syndromes.

Answer to Question 15

B

The purpose of the pentose phosphate pathway is to generate NADPH and pentose sugars.

NADPH is required for many biosynthetic reactions (e.g. fatty acid synthesis), as well as for maintenance of reduced glutathione levels and erythrocyte structure.

The pentose sugars, ribose and deoxyribose, are components of nucleotides, and hence of DNA and RNA.

In the first stage of the pentose phosphate pathway, both NADPH and ribose-5-phosphate are generated. If the cell's requirement for NADPH exceeds that for pentose sugars, the ribose phophate is recycled back to glycolytic intermediates.

Answer to Question 16

A

Arginine is positively charged at physiological pH. The pK of an amino acid is the pH at which 50% of its side chains are protonated: at lower pH the proportion that are protonated rises, those of arginine (pK 12.5) being almost completely protonated at physiological pH.

Histidine is another amino acid that can accept protons at physiological pH and become positively charged. Its pK is 6.0, and is modified by the local environment. This is much closer to physiological pH, enabling histidine to act as a reversible proton carrier, e.g. in haemoglobin. Dibasic amino acids with positively charged side chains are cystine, ornithine, arginine and lysine. In cystinuria a defect of the dibasic amino acid transporter in the renal tubule leads to excess quantities of all of these amino acids being present in the urine, when cystine rises to concentrations that are insoluble, leading to the formation of cystine stones.

Answer to Question 17

C

Humans can synthesise 11 of the basic set of 20 amino acids. The rest must be obtained from the diet: histidine, isoleucine, leucine, lysine, methionine, phenylalanine, threonine, tryptophan and valine are therefore known as 'essential' amino acids.

Synthesis of those amino acids that can be made proceeds as follows: the carbon skeleton usually arises from metabolic intermediates such as oxaloacetate and pyruvate; amino acids are donated by other amino acids in transamination reactions; extra amino groups are sometimes derived from ammonia after first being incorporated into glutamate by the enzyme glutamate dehydrogenase.

Answer to Question 18

B

Alpha helices are one of the secondary structures found within proteins. They are generally right handed, and are stabilised by hydrogen bonding parallel to the helical axis. The side chains project outwards, and determine the interactions of the helix with neighbouring structures.

Transmembrane domains are mostly hydrophobic, as they lie within a lipid environment.

Proline residues form kinks in the backbone and are not compatible within an alpha-helical structure.

Collagen has a helical form that is very different from an alpha-helix. It has a high proportion of proline and hydroxyproline, and nearly every third residue is a glycine. The helix of collagen is more open than that of an alpha-helix and is not stabilised by hydrogen bonding within the helix. Rather, three helical strands are wound around each other to form a superhelix, with hydrogen bonds between the strands.

Answer to Question 19

A

Protein synthesis is catalysed by ribosomes, begins with an initiator methionine, and proceeds by the addition of further amino acids to the free carboxyl terminus.

The mRNA is translated in the 5′ to 3′ direction and is read in groups of 3 bases, which are known as codons. Amino acids are carried to the growing chain by transfer (t)RNAs. Binding of the correct tRNA, and hence the addition of the correct next amino acid, is ensured by the matching between the codon on the mRNA and the anti-codon on the tRNA. Several amino acids are specified by a number of codons, and in these cases the tRNA can bind even if the third position in the codon does not match that in the anti-codon. This is known as the 'wobble' position. Whether a wobble is allowed at the third position is determined by the residue at the first position of the codon.

The poly-A tail can influence the initiation of translation via the binding of special poly-A binding proteins, but it is not the place at which the ribosome is assembled, which occurs at the Cap structure at the 5′ end. It may be involved in mRNA stability.

Ricin is a toxin from castor beans, which inactivates ribosomes by catalysing the removal of a single adenosine from ribosomal RNA: it is an inhibitor of translation, not of transcription.

Answer to Question 20

D

Gluconeogenesis is effectively the reverse of glycolysis, enabling the synthesis of glucose from metabolic intermediates, such as pyruvate. It uses alternative enzymes for some reactions to control the relative rates of the forward and reverse pathways, allowing cells to adapt to their specific needs.

Acetyl CoA, produced by beta oxidation or from ketone bodies, cannot be used as a substrate, because it cannot be reconverted to pyruvate.

Lactate is a reduced form of pyruvate, and is converted back to pyruvate by lactate dehydrogenase in the liver. Alanine is the transaminated form of pyruvate, and is therefore another substrate for gluconeogenesis. Amino acids, such as glutamine and glutamate, feed into the citric acid cycle at the level of alpha-ketoglutarate, which is subsequently converted to oxaloacetic acid, another starting point of gluconeogenesis. Glycerol, derived from breakdown of triacylglycerols, is a substrate for gluconeogenesis.

Cell Biology

Answer to Question 21

B

Steroids bind to cytosolic receptors, which leads them to dimerize with translocation of the ligand–receptor complex to the nucleus. The response to receptor activation is mediated by specific binding of these complexes to promoter or enhancer elements of genes and modulation of gene transcription.

Answer to Question 22

A

Anti-epileptic drugs which stimulate GABA receptors directly, or indirectly by increasing GABA levels, include sodium valproate, benzodiazepines and vigabatrin. Stimulation of GABA receptors triggers opening of associated Cl^- channels and influx of Cl^- into the cell. The Cl^- influx hyperpolarises cell membranes, reducing the likelihood that voltage-gated Na^+ channels will open, hence preventing Na^+ influx into the cell and stabilising the cell membrane.

Answer to Question 23

D

There are two mechanisms for cell death: necrosis, which is a passive response to injury, and apoptosis, a mechanism of programmed cell death for removing excess cells produced during development or for removing cells that are functionally impaired, deficient or abnormal. Apoptosis can result from multiple stimuli or the removal of survival factors such as hormones or growth factors.

p53 is an important initiator following cellular injury. The process of apoptosis involves a rapid and sustained increase in intracellular calcium that triggers endonuclease activation, leading to cleavage of DNA into fragments of about 180 base pairs. These can be detected as a DNA 'ladder' on gel electrophoresis.

Answer to Question 24

E

The cell cycle has five phases:

1. GO – most cells in normal adult tissues are in this quiescent phase
2. G1 – the first gap phase that occurs prior to the initiation of DNA synthesis and is a period of commitment that separates M and S phases as cells prepare for DNA duplication
3. S – the phase of DNA synthesis
4. G2 – the second gap phase that occurs after DNA synthesis and before mitosis. Errors in DNA are repaired during this phase
5. M – mitosis, which completes the cell cycle

Answer to Question 25

C

Na/K-ATPase transporters are found in all living cells in the body. They are comprised of alpha and beta subunits, the alpha subunit containing regions that coordinate cation transport and regions that bind and hydrolyse ATP, releasing energy to drive the transport of three sodium ions out of the cell for every two potassium ions imported. Action of the pump, which is inhibited by digoxin, maintains the cell's resting membrane potential.

Answer to Question 26

A

The main cellular source of TNF is the macrophage. The use of biological agents that inhibit TNF in the treatment of Crohn's disease and inflammatory arthritides has emphasised the importance of TNF in inflammatory and apoptotic pathways. The TNFα gene is located on chromosome 6p21 in the middle of the MHC. It is closely linked to neighbouring genes that encode lymphotoxin A and lymphotoxin B. TNF polymorphisms have been associated with a number of different autoimmune diseases, including type I diabetes mellitus, multiple sclerosis and rheumatoid arthritis, but it remains to be established whether the genetic predisposition operates through variations in function and/or expression of TNF

or through other linked genes that lie linked within the MHC region. There are multiple single nucleotide polymorphisms across the TNF gene and some haplotypes are associated with variation in levels of expression. Both genetic and functional studies support an association of TNF with survival in septic shock and in the susceptibility to cerebral malaria.

Answer to Question 27

C

Nitric oxide lacks a classical receptor and has a unique mechanism of action. It diffuses freely into cells where it activates a soluble cytosolic form of guanylate cyclase, causing an elevation in cGMP. Nitrovasodilator drugs in clinical use, e.g. GTN, act as exogenous sources of nitric oxide, producing relaxation of blood vessels via increases in intracellular cGMP in vascular smooth muscle cells.

Answer to Question 28

D

Signal transduction within a cell commonly results in phosphorylation and activation of key intracellular proteins such as ion channels, enzymes or transporters that are the effectors of biological responses. These phosphorylation reactions often occur at serine or threonine residues and are catalysed by kinases, which are themselves activated by the binding of intracellular messengers. Protein kinase A is activated by cAMP, protein kinase G by cGMP, and protein kinase C by diacylglycerol.

Answer to Question 29

E

The NaCl co-transporter is located in the distal tubule where it contributes to the reabsorption of about 10% of the filtered load of sodium. Thiazide diuretics cause a natriuresis by blocking the actions of this co-transporter and hence reducing the amount of sodium and chloride reabsorbed in the distal tubule. Mutations causing loss of function of the NaCl co-transporter cause Gitelman's syndrome, the commonest monogenic cause of hypokalaemia in adults.

Answer to Question 30

A

The resting potential of most cells (about −80 mV) is determined by the fact that most channels open in the cell membrane are K channels and the intracellular potassium concentration (140 mmol/l) is much higher than the extracellular (4 mmol/l). Depolarisation of the cell membrane triggers rapid opening of voltage-gated sodium channels, causing a flux of sodium into the cell down its concentration gradient (extracellular 140 mmol/l, intracellular 10 mmol/l) and generating the rapid depolarisation of the action potential.

Immunology and Immunosuppression

Answer to Question 31
E

The T cell receptor gene is rearranged to give each receptor, and hence each T cell, a unique specificity – just like antibody genes. Also like antibody genes, each T cell only has one kind of receptor – this is known as allelic exclusion. There are two chains, alpha and beta, and these are always found with CD3, and either CD4 or CD8 (for T helper and T cytotoxic cells respectively).

Answer to Question 32
E

Cyclosporin and tacrolimus are both calcineurin inhibitors – the former binding to calcineurin as a complex with cyclophillin A, and the latter as a complex with FKBP12. Rapamycin also binds to FKBP12, but this complex inhibits cell proliferation by binding to the mammalian target of rapamycin (mTOR). Mycophenolate mofetil, not azathioprine, acts through inosine monophosphate dehydrogenase inhibition.

Answer to Question 33
D

All of these cells develop in the bone marrow, except for T cells, which develop in the thymus.

Answer to Question 34
E

Cytolytic granules contain membrane perturbing molecules that allow fusion of the killer cell with the target cell: these include perforins and granulysin. Fusion allows the release of granule contents into the target cell, and molecules such as granzymes induce apoptosis.

The membrane attack complex is part of the complement pathway and is not found in cytolytic granules.

Answer to Question 35
D

X-linked agammaglobulinaemia usually presents by around 6 months of age.

IVIG contains low levels of IgA and is not a suitable treatment for IgA deficiency.

Chronic granulomatous disease is due to a range of neutrophil defects that result in an impaired respiratory burst. Chemotaxis and phagocytosis are unimpaired.

Despite an impaired ability to mount normal antibody responses, patients with CVID are predisposed to diseases such as pernicious anaemia and autoimmune thyroid disease.

Defects in terminal (not classical) pathway complement components predispose to Neisserial infections.

Answer to Question 36
D

T-helper cells are distinguished by the presence of CD4 on their surface and their ability to recognise peptides presented on MHC class II molecules. Their functions include promoting delayed-type hypersensitivity reactions, characterised by monocyte recruitment, and providing help for B-cell antibody production.

Cytotoxic T cells have CD8 on their surface and recognise peptide presented on MHC class I molecules.

Answer to Question 37
B

CD4 cells differentiate into two main groups called Th1 and Th2. The former are important for activating macrophages, the latter for activating B cells and stimulating humoral immunity. Cytokines secreted by Th2 cells include Il 4, 5, 6, 10 and 13. Cytokines secreted by Th 1 cells include IFN-gamma, Il2 and TGF beta.

Answer to Question 38
D

The innate immune system is available the first time that a pathogen is encountered, does not require previous exposure to that pathogen, and is not modified by repeated exposure to the pathogen over time. It provides the first line of defence and reacts more quickly than the adaptive immune system. Pattern recognition receptors such as toll-like receptors and scavenger receptors distinguish self from non-self. Many types of leukocyte are involved, including all of those listed above with the exception of B cells.

The adaptive immune system comprises B and T lymphocytes. Clones of B and T cells have antigen receptors recognising specific antigens. Some of the cells of the innate immune system can also present antigen to T cells of the adaptive immune system.

Answer to Question 39

D

All of these are soluble complement inhibitors, except CD59 which is membrane bound. Other membrane bound complement inhibitors include complement receptor 1, decay accelerating factor, and membrane cofactor protein.

Answer to Question 40

A

The processing pathway for class I typically involves newly synthesized proteins being degraded by proteosomes, and transported into the endoplasmic reticulum by TAP proteins for loading onto class I.

For class II presentation, exogenous antigens are taken up and degraded, with the invariant chain stabilising class II until it is loaded with peptide. The invariant chain therefore plays a role in class II processing but is not structurally related to class II.

The MHC class III region encodes molecules that include complement proteins and tumour necrosis factor (TNF), which are not functionally or structurally related to class I or II.

Anatomy

Answer to Question 41

C

In the petrous temporal bone the facial nerve produces three branches:

1. The greater petrosal nerve, which transmits preganglionic parasympathetic fibres to the sphenopaletine ganglion, whose postganglionic fibres supply the lacrimal gland and the glands in the nasal cavity
2. The nerve to stapedius
3. Parasympathetic fibres to the submandibular and sublingual glands and taste fibres from the anterior two-thirds of the tongue.

Answer to Question 42

B

From the auditory nuclei in the brain stem impulses are transmitted to the inferior colliculus and medial geniculate body of both sides through the trapezoid body and the lateral lemnisci. From there they reach the auditory cortex via the auditory radiations.

Answer to Question 43

B

About 75% of the blood supply to the liver comes from the portal vein, which is formed by the union of superior mesenteric and splenic veins.

Inside the liver, blood from the portal vein and from the hepatic artery flows through the tortuous capillaries called sinusoids. The venous outflow to the inferior vena cava from the liver is via the hepatic veins and obstruction to this outflow causes Budd–Chiari syndrome.

The normal portal pressure is about 5–8 mm Hg: in portal hypertension it rises above 10–12 mm Hg.

Answer to Question 44

E

The right and left hepatic ducts join together to form the common hepatic duct, which in turn is joined by the cystic duct to form the bile duct in the free border of the lesser omentum. The bile duct then passes behind the first part of the duodenum and the head of the pancreas, joins with the pancreatic duct to form the ampulla of Vater, and opens into the second part of the duodenum on its posteromedial wall on the papilla of Vater.

The papilla is 10 cms distal to the pylorus.

The sphincter of Oddi surrounds the ampulla as well as the ends of the common bile duct and pancreatic ducts.

Answer to Question 45

B

The apical pleura and lung project about 3–4 cms above the inner aspect of the clavicle, where they are related to the subclavian vessels and the brachial plexus: hence a chest radiograph to exclude pneumothorax is warranted following subclavian vein cannulation.

The oblique fissure lies between the upper and lower lobes. The horizontal fissure, often seen on a plain radiograph, demarcates the middle lobe from the upper lobe on the right side.

The lower border of the lung extends up to the tenth rib at the back and the pleura up to the twelfth, hence the lung and pleura overlaps the liver, kidney and spleen.

Answer to Question 46
D

The apex beat is the lowest and most lateral cardiac pulsation in the precordium. It is felt normally in the fourth or fifth intercostal space in the midclavicular line but shifts to the anterior axillary line when lying on the left side. It may be found further laterally in left ventricular enlargement, also (less commonly) in conditions producing lower mediastinal shift. The apex is often impalpable in obese patients and in those with emphysema, pericardial effusion and/or pleural effusion.

A tapping apex beat, as felt in mitral stenosis, is a sudden brief pulsation. A heaving beat (forceful and sustained impulse) is due to pressure overload as in hypertension and aortic stenosis. A thrusting (forceful but not sustained) beat is caused by volume overload as in mitral or aortic regurgitation.

Answer to Question 47
B

There are usually four parathyroid glands, lying in the substance of the thyroid gland posteriorly. They are developed from the third and fourth branchial pouches, the third pouch derivatives descending further down to form the inferior pair, with those derived from the fourth pouch becoming the superior parathyroids.

The arterial supply of the parathyroids is mostly from the inferior thyroid arteries: this may be compromised during thyroidectomy, the incidence of hypocalcaemia being 30–40%.

Answer to Question 48
A

The right bronchus is shorter, wider and more vertical than the left one. It divides into three main lobar bronchi to ventilate the three lobes of the right lung. The left lung usually has only two lobes.

The bronchial walls contain cartilage, smooth muscle and submucosal glands. Bronchioles are tubes less than 2 mm in diameter and are devoid of cartilage or submucosal glands.

Answer to Question 49
E

Ptosis is caused by paralysis of the levator palpebrae superioris muscle, innervated by the oculomotor nerve as well as the sympathetics. Ptosis therefore is a characteristic of 3rd nerve paralysis and Horner's syndrome. The orbicularis oculi, which is essential for blinking, is supplied by the facial nerve.

The suspensory ligament anchors the lens to the ciliary body. Its tension flattens the lens. In accommodation the ligament is slackened by the contraction of the ciliary muscle, making the lens more spherical.

The refractory index of the lens is about 15 dioptres and is more than that of vitreous and aqueous humours.

The aqueous humour is produced by the ciliary processes. Choroid plexuses are in the ventricles of the brain, not in the eye.

Aqueous humour, produced in the posterior chamber, is absorbed into the Canal of Shlemm, which is a vein at the iridocorneal angle of the anterior chamber.

Answer to Question 50
D

The testis develops in the L2–L3 vertebral region and drags its vascular supply, lymphatics and nerve supply from this region to the scrotum. Testicular pain may therefore radiate to the loin and renal pain may be referred to the scrotum.

The lymphatics of the testis drain into the para-aortic nodes.

The epididymis lies on the posterolateral aspect of the testis and the ductus deferens continues from the tail of the epididymis into the spermatic cord.

Physiology

Answer to Question 51
A

At any given time in the cardiac cycle, the membrane potential is chiefly determined by the conductance of the membrane to a number of key ions. When the conductance to a particular ion increases, the membrane potential moves towards the 'reversal potential' of that ion, which is the potential at which the electromotive force to move that ion across the membrane exactly balances the concentration gradient. Because sodium and calcium concentrations are considerably higher outside the cell than inside, the reversal potentials for these ions are positive, i.e. these ions act as a depolarizing influence. The concentration gradient for potassium operates in the opposite way and this ion is a major repolarization force.

At rest the only ion with significant trans-membrane conductance is potassium, and the resting membrane potential therefore sits close to the potassium reversal potential, at about –80 mV with respect to the extracellular fluid. When the membrane potential is driven less negative by interaction with nearby depolarized cells, voltage-activated channels are opened, which greatly increase trans-membrane conductance of sodium, depolarizing the cell (phase 0 of the action potential). At potentials around 0 mV, slow calcium channels are activated, contributing to the maintenance of depolarization at the plateau of the action potential (phase 2).

Answer to Question 52

B

The functional residual volume is the volume of air left after a quiet expiration and is approximately 3 L. The dead space in an adult is about a 150 mL and represents the volume of inspired air that does not reach the alveoli. Residual volume is the gas that remains in the chest after maximal expiration.

The phrenic nerve supplies the diaphragm and is derived from the C3, C4 and C5 nerve roots.

Answer to Question 53

C

The main stimulus for aldosterone production by the adrenal gland is angiotensin 2, but production is also stimulated by hyperkalaemia. A high level of aldosterone leads to hypokalaemia. The main site of action of aldosterone is the collecting duct, where it binds to a cytoplasmic mineralocorticoid receptor and leads to increased numbers and activity of apical ENaC (sodium) and ROMK (potassium) channels, also of the basolateral Na/K-ATPase. The effect of aldosterone is to simultaneously increase reabsorption of sodium and increase excretion of potassium by the collecting duct. Spironolactone binds to the cytoplasmic mineralocorticoid receptor, preventing the action of aldosterone, and amiloride blocks the ENaC channel. Both therefore reduce the reabsorption of sodium and reduce the excretion of potassium, i.e. they are potassium sparing diuretics.

Answer to Question 54

C

Intravenous calcium gluconate (10 ml of 10%, repeated as necessary) is the first line treatment of severe hyperkalaemia: it acts to 'stabilise' the cardiac membranes within 1–2 mins but has no effect on the serum potassium concentration.

Both glucose (50 ml of 50%) and insulin (10–20 units of a rapidly acting preparation) or a beta-agonist can reduce the serum potassium concentration by 1–2 mmol/l over 20–30 min. They do so by directly stimulating cellular Na/K-ATPase, which drives potassium into cells.

Calcium resonium (which cannot be given intravenously) acts as an ion exchange resin in the gut, exchanging potassium for calcium, which is then excreted. It takes at least 4–6 hr to have any effect and is therefore not an emergency treatment for hyperkalaemia. Peritoneal dialysis is similarly slow in its effect: haemodialysis is the preferred form of renal replacement therapy in the patient with severe hyperkalaemia.

Answer to Question 55

C

The renal clearance of any substance is calculated from the formula: Urine concentration × Urine volume / Plasma concentration.

Clearance of a substance can be used to estimate glomerular filtration rate (GFR) if the substance is:
- Freely filtered at the glomerulus
- Not secreted or reabsorbed by the renal tubules
- Not metabolised in any way by the kidney

In clinical practice the substance most commonly used to measure GFR by calculation of clearance is creatinine, which is a low molecular weight product (MW 113) of creatine and phosphocreatine catabolism in muscle.

Answer to Question 56

E

90–99.9% of sodium filtered at the glomerulus is reabsorbed by the renal tubule, 75% of it in the proximal tubule.

In the proximal tubule sodium enters the cells from the lumen on several different types of carrier, including the sodium-hydrogen exchanger (NHE-3). The main methods by which sodium enters tubular cells in the rest of the nephron are as follows: in the thick ascending limb of Henle's loop via the Na/K/2Cl co-transporter (the site of action of frusemide and other loop diuretics); in the distal convoluted tubule via the thiazide sensitive sodium-chloride co-transporter (TSC); and in the collecting duct via the epithelial sodium channel (ENaC) (the site of action of amiloride).

The main 'metabolic engine' driving sodium reabsorption along the renal tubule is the Na/K-ATPase located along the basolateral border of tubular cells.

In the collecting duct aldosterone binds to a cytoplasmic mineralocorticoid receptor and stimulates increased numbers and activity of apical ENaC and potassium channels (ROMK), and of basolateral Na/K-ATPase by direct and indirect effects.

Answer to Question 57

C

The myofibril is made up of thick and thin filaments. Every thick filament is made up of about 300 myosin molecules. Each thin filament has a tropomyosin backbone around which are wound two helical chains of actin. Troponin T binds the whole troponin complex to tropomyosin; troponin I inhibits contraction; troponin C binding regulates troponin I.

Answer to Question 58

A

The R wave of the ECG occurs just before mitral valve closure and therefore marks the end of cardiac diastole.

Answer to Question 59

B

$BP = CO \times TPR$

Answer to Question 60

D

Small arteries and arterioles are the major contributors to peripheral resistance because resistance and vessel radius are related according to Laplace's law, which states that resistance is proportional to the fourth power of the radius (r^4). This means that a very small change in radius causes a very large increase in resistance.

Answer to Question 61

B

Nitric oxide is synthesised from L-arginine by the action of nitric oxide synthase, producing L-citrulline in the process. Nitric oxide has a half-life of only a few seconds and is produced continuously by the vascular endothelium. Several physiological/pharmacological agents stimulate nitric oxide release, including acetyl choline, bradykinin and substance P.

Answer to Question 62

E

Cholecystokinin is released from the jejunal mucosa in response to fat. It is a potent inhibitor of gastric motility and secretion, causes contraction of the gall bladder (emptying bile into the duodenal lumen, where it acts as a detergent, breaking the fat into micelles), and it stimulates the exocrine pancreas to produce proteases (trypsin and chymotrypsin), lipases and amylases.

Pancreatic secretion of bicarbonate, which neutralises the acidic gastric effluent to provide optimum pH for the function of pancreatic enzymes, is stimulated by secretin.

Answer to Question 63

A

Bilirubin is formed when the ring structure of haem is broken open by microsomal haem oxygenase. It is then bound to albumin, transferred to the liver, where it is conjugated, allowing secretion into bile as mono- or di-glucuronide. In the distal intestine, conjugate bilirubin is deconjugated and reduced to a series of sterco- and uro-bilinogens that give the faeces their typical colour. Some colourless urobilinogen is normally absorbed from the colon and undergoes enterohepatic circulation, with a small amount being excreted in the urine. This cannot happen if biliary obstruction prevents bile from entering the gut.

Answer to Question 64

E

The sodium-potassium (Na/K) ATPase pump transports three sodium ions out of the cell for every two potassium ions transported in. Thus at rest potassium ions are predominantly intracellular and sodium ions extracellular. Each ion tends to diffuse down its concentration gradient, but only to a point where electrochemical balance is maintained. If the cell membrane were permeable only to sodium, then this equilibrium resting membrane potential would be about +60 mV (inside positive); if permeable only to potassium it would be about –95 mV. At its resting state the cell membrane is permeable to potassium ions but not to sodium, hence the resting membrane potential is about –80 mV.

Answer to Question 65

D

An inhibitory postsynaptic potential results in increased permeability to only potassium and chloride ions. As the equilibrium potential of both these ions is negative, hyperpolarisation results.

An excitatory postsynaptic potential results in increased permeability to all ions. This causes a small depolarisation as a result of net influx of sodium ions. There is no great increase in the flux of potassium ions the resting membrane is already relatively permeable to them and the resting membrane potential is not very different from the equilibrium potential for potassium.

Answer to Question 66

D

The axon terminal of a motor nerve contains about 300,000 vesicles of the neurotransmitter acetylcholine. When an action potential arrives at the nerve terminal, about 300 vesicles are released into the synaptic cleft. Acetycholine diffuses across the cleft and binds to the postsynaptic nicotinic acetylcholine receptor, triggering an action potential across the muscle membrane. Within 1 ms most acetycholine is destroyed by acetylcholinesterase, which is found at high concentration at the motor end-plate.

Answer to Question 67

D

Growth hormone has direct 'anti-insulin' effects, but its anabolic actions are mediated through insulin-like growth factor 1 (IGF1), which is produced by the liver. The amount of IGF1 produced depends on the well-being of the animal: less is produced in response to growth hormone if food is absent or if the immune system is activated.

The large circulating pool of IGF1 is bound to high affinity binding proteins, mainly IGF-binding protein 3 (IGFBP3). When this is proteolytically cleaved its affinity for IGF1 is reduced, releasing IGF1 to bind to its cell surface receptors.

Answer to Question 68

A

Aldosterone is produced by the zona glomerulosa under the regulation of the renin-angiotensin system. The zona fasciculata produces glucocorticoids (cortisol), the zona reticularis androgens, and the adrenal medulla catecholamines.

Answer to Question 69

E

Increase in blood osmolality, sensed by osmoreceptors in the organ vasculosum of the lamina terminalis (OVLT), is responsible for modulation of ADH secretion to control plasma tonicity. However, intravascular volume depletion, nausea and pain are all much more powerful stimuli for ADH release than alteration in plasma tonicity, meaning that very high levels of ADH are expected after surgery. Patients are unable to excrete a water load normally immediately postoperatively and profound (and deadly) hyponatraemia can result if large quantities of 5% dextrose are given intravenously.

Answer to Question 70

C

In cells of the proximal tubule, distal tubule and collecting duct glutamine is converted to glutamate and then to α-ketoglutarate, each of these steps releasing an ammonium ion that is excreted in the urine. Metabolism of α-ketoglutarate subsequently releases two bicarbonate ions that are reabsorbed into the circulation.

Clinical Pharmacology

Answer to Question 71

C

Convulsions should be treated immediately in the usual way, without waiting for confirmation of the theophylline level.

Theophylline is metabolised by the CYP450 enzymes in the liver. Erythromycin inhibits CYP450 enzymes and increases the half-life of theophylline and hence plasma theophylline concentrations, which may lead to toxicity. By contrast, phenytoin induces CYP450 enzymes, which will decrease the half-life of theophylline and may lead to inadequate therapeutic levels.

Theophylline toxicity is more likely in the elderly due to age-related reduction in the rate of its metabolism, but it can occur at any age.

Theophylline is an example of a drug with a NARROW therapeutic range. It is recommended that plasma theophylline levels be maintained between 10 and 20 mg/l.

Answer to Question 72

B

Bendrofluazide tends to cause hypokalaemia.

The other drugs listed may cause hyperkalaemia, although this is not usually clinically significant when used alone at therapeutic doses. The development of significant drug-induced hyperkalaemia is more likely when more than one of these agents is used in combination, or if the patient has co-existing renal impairment.

Answer to Question 73

D

Drugs can cause haemolytic anaemia by a variety of mechanisms. Penicillin binds covalently to the red blood cell membranes; rifampicin causes immune complex association with red blood cell membranes leading to complement activation; methyldopa and mefenamic acid may induce the formation of autoantibodies against components of red blood cells. Ranitidine is not reported to cause haemolytic anaemia.

Answer to Question 74

B

The anti-thyroid drug carbimazole causes neutropenia in 1 in 800 patients. The Committee of Safety of Medicines (CSM) advise that patients taking carbimazole should be asked to report any symptoms or signs suggestive of infection immediately, especially sore throat. A white blood count should be performed if there is any clinical suspicion of infection, and if there is clinical or laboratory evidence of neutropenia the carbimazole should be stopped promptly.

Answer to Question 75

C

Digoxin is the most likely cause of his gynaecomastia. This side effect is more common with longer-term use and may be unilateral or bilateral. Important differential diagnoses to consider include male breast cancer, liver disease, testicular tumours and hyperthyroidism.

Other drugs that can cause gynaecomastia include oestrogens, spironolactone, cimetidine, verapamil and nifedipine. The gynaecomastia usually improves on stopping the drug or reducing the dose.

Answer to Question 76

E

Dystonic reactions are well-recognized with dopamine receptor antagonists.

They occur shortly after starting therapy, particularly in girls and young women as well as the elderly. The problem usually subsides within 24 hours following cessation of treatment and can be treated with procyclidine 5–10 mg IM (an antimuscarinic).

Answer to Question 77

E

Amiodarone is an iodine rich molecule that resembles T4. A daily dose of 200 mg generates 7 mg free iodine, compared with the WHO optimal intake of 0.15–0.3 mg/day.

This high iodine load blocks further iodide uptake and hormone synthesis by the thyroid, and it also blocks conversion of T4 to T3 and affects the pituitary thyroid axis. The following changes in thyroid function tests can occur within 3 months of starting amiodarone and are not indicative of thyroid disease: increase in TSH up to 20 mU/L, increase in T4 to upper limit of normal range, and decreased T3 levels. The diagnosis of hypothyrodism should be based on clinical assessment, together with the following features: high TSH of > 20 mU/l, low free T4, low T3. Treatment is with thyroxine, aiming for free T4 levels close to the upper limit of the normal range.

Answer to Question 78

C

Suxamethonium is a depolarising neuromuscular blocking agent that is metabolised by plasma pseudocholinesterases. Approximately 1/2500 individuals have deficiency of this enzyme, resulting in prolonged neuromuscular blockade if suxamethonium is given. Management is by prolonged ventilation until the action of the drug wears off. Relatives of affected patients should be screened.

Answer to Question 79

E

Ezetimibe is the first of a novel class of drugs for the treatment of hyperlipidaemia whose main action is to specifically prevent cholesterol absorption from the small intestine. It typically reduces LDL-cholesterol by about 20%, triglycerides by up to 5% and raises HDL-cholesterol by approximately 5%. It does not inhibit the absorption of fat-soluble vitamins, unlike the anion-exchange resins (e.g. colestyramine). Ezetimibe can be safely co-administered with statins and is currently licensed for use in combination with a statin in patients who fail to reach desired lipid profiles or as monotherapy in patients intolerant of a statin. There is no increased risk of myopathy with ezetimibe prescription.

Answer to Question 80

C

Memantine is the first licensed NMDA receptor antagonist for the management of moderate to severe Alzheimer's disease. It has small benefit in reducing deterioration in patients with this condition, but little evidence for use in other types of dementia. Several drug interactions are known:

• NMDA antagonists (e.g. ketamine, amantadine) – can precipitate psychosis
• Dopamine agonists – effects enhanced
• Barbiturates and neuroleptics – effects reduced
• Drugs excreted by cationic transporters in the kidney (e.g. ranitidine, quinine, nicotine) – excretion reduced leading to higher plasma concentrations.

Answer to Question 81

C

Insulin glargine is a long-acting insulin analogue, produced by modifying the chemical structure of insulin. This gives it a smooth, prolonged absorption profile with no peaks. As such, it is a long-acting agent, suitable for providing a basal level of insulin that attempts to mimic the normal physiological state. Its smooth profile reduces the risk of hypoglycaemia, and when given at night it provides good control of the fasting blood glucose. Unlike crystalline suspensions, insulin glargine does not need to be mixed thoroughly prior to injection, making it easier to use.

Answer to Question 82

B

Low-dose diuretics are accepted as the first-line treatment for hypertension in the elderly and appear to confer greater benefit than beta-adrenergic receptor antagonists in this population. Treatment of isolated systolic hypertension in the elderly with the long-acting calcium channel blocker nitrendipine has been shown to reduce stroke and adverse cardiovascular outcome. Calcium channel blockers may therefore be suitable when diurectics are not tolerated, ineffective or contra-indicated.

Answer to Question 83

C

Calcium-channel blockers (CCBs) and diuretics appear to be the most effective antihypertensives in Afro-Caribbeans. Diuretics have the disadvantage that they commonly cause impotence. Short-acting CCBs do not provide prolonged blood pressure control, can cause reflex tachycardia, and may be associated with higher mortality. A long-acting CCB should be the first-line drug of choice, ideally a once-daily agent that provides smooth 24-hour BP control, e.g. Nifedipine LA 30 mg od or Amlodipine 5 mg od.

ACE (angiotensin-converting enzyme) inhibitors and beta-receptor antagonists are less effective in Afro-Caribbeans, probably because the renin-angiotensin-aldosterone system is usually suppressed in this ethnic group such that drugs that act by suppressing the RAA system are unlikely to be effective.

Answer to Question 84

A

All of these are recognized treatments for status epilepticus. First-line treatment should be with intravenous benzodiazepine, with lorazepam preferred to diazepam because of its longer duration of action. Fosphenytoin is the preferred second-line treatment (phenytoin if this is not available). Phenobarbitone is one of several agents that can be used as third-line treatment, but seek specialist advice if first and second-line treatments are ineffective.

Answer to Question 85

B

The potency of a drug relates to the amount of drug needed to produce a given effect. An equivalent diuresis to that seen with drugs A and B is produced with a considerably smaller dose of C, which is therefore more potent.

Efficacy relates to the maximal response that can be produced by the drug when taken at high dose. Despite increasing the dose, drug C is unable to produce an equivalent maximal diuresis to that obtained with drugs A or B, it is thus of lower efficacy.

The potency of a drug is not often of importance but can become significant if the drug has low solubility and has to be packaged or delivered in such a way that space is limited. Examples might include metered dose aerosols or depot injections.

Statistics, Epidemiology, Clinical Trials, Meta-analyses and Evidence-based Medicine

Answer to Question 86

A

Forest plots are most commonly used in meta-analyses as a concise and elegant way of presenting information from many individual trials, allowing a convenient visual comparison of the separate trial results together with a synthesis of the data.

The horizontal lines emerging from the squares represent confidence intervals. Larger studies have narrower confidence intervals, hence the largest squares are typically associated with the smallest horizontal lines.

Answer to Question 87

B

Most trials evaluate just one treatment. This does not have to be so: factorial trials test two or more treatments simultaneously.

A famous example of a factorial trial was the ISIS-2 study in which comparison was made between placebo and each of two drugs, streptokinase and aspirin. Patients with suspected myocardial infarction were randomised to receive IV streptokinase alone, aspirin alone, both active drugs, or double placebo. The trial showed that each of the drugs produced about a 25% reduction in mortality, also that their effects were additive.

Answer to Question 88

A

Interpreting the sensitivity and specificity of a test depends on what you are using it for.

The poor specificity of this test means that it would be inappropriate to use it as reason for telling people they have HIV infection; in the at-risk population over 50% diagnosed positive will not have the disease. By contrast, the balance of risk is different in screening blood for HIV, where the risk of missing a positive case far outweighs the risk of discarding some blood units unnecessarily, and similarly in looking for bowel cancer.

The test would also potentially be appropriate in screening for head lice where the disease is not serious but you do not want to miss cases and the treatment is simple and safe.

Predictive value depends as much on prevalence of a condition as the sensitivity. The positive predictive value in young patients means most army recruits with a positive test would be false-positive, with more being false-positive than true-positive, but since very few are likely to have heart disease a preliminary screening test with a positive predictive value of 48% would be a reasonable test to use.

Answer to Question 89

D

With a cohort study you start with two (or more) groups with different exposures. This could be exposure to an occupational hazard, or to different drugs or different infections. You then follow them over time to see whether, and when, they develop an outcome (in medicine usually a disease, complication or death). Cohort studies are therefore very good for investigating the effects of rare exposures, as you set the exposure. If the outcome is rare it is unlikely enough cases will occur in the follow-up time to draw any conclusions, so they are not good for rare outcomes.

Unlike other study designs cohort studies follow individuals over time, so are particularly good for measuring incidence of a disease. They are not the best study design for measuring prevalence of a disease in a population (cross-sectional studies are very well designed for this).

Answer to Question 90

E

It is only ethical to conduct a clinical trial if it is capable of detecting a meaningful difference between two treatments to guide future practice. If a trial is underpowered it cannot detect a statistically significant difference. It is therefore mandatory to do a proper power calculation before exposing patients to a clinical trial.

The rather daunting formal definition of a type I error means that a study falsely (but not deliberately) appears to find a difference between two groups which has actually arisen by chance alone. The conventional cut-off of $p < 0.05$ will arise by chance alone one time in twenty. As many thousands of studies are published every month, type I errors are not rare.

A type II error is formally where the null hypothesis is falsely accepted. To claim two treatments are 'equivalent' requires huge numbers, and most studies are underpowered (too small) to reliably rule out a small difference between one treatment and another.

Most published studies are small enough that type I and type II errors are a real possibility, and examples are published in good journals every week.

Answer to Question 91

D

The principle of a crossover design is that a patient has one drug or treatment, then a washout period, and then another drug, and the effect is compared between the two in a single individual. For this reason it is a good study design for treatment of chronic conditions, but not appropriate for acute conditions.

It is just as easy (or difficult) to randomize and double-blind as for other study designs.

Because each person is acting as their own control, it is usually possible to use smaller numbers to get the same power.

Answer to Question 92

B

Case-control studies compare exposures of interest in cases and controls. Two of their great strengths is that they can be used with rare diseases (because cases are pre-selected), and can examine multiple risk-factors (exposures).

They are not good at identifying rare exposures. If the question is whether or not a rare exposure causes a disease then the appropriate design is a cohort study, where one group with the particular exposure of interest is compared with a control group without that exposure.

The greatest difficulty in designing case-control studies is selection of an appropriate control group, and poor control selection often makes otherwise well-conducted studies uninterpretable.

Answer to Question 93

B

Looking at a set of data plotted out on a graph is a good way of determining whether or not it is skewed. There is no such thing as a 'skew test'.

There are few absolutes in statistics, but one is that skewed data should never be described by the mean, as it will lead to misleading distortions.

Chi-squared is for categorical data.

It is possible to use Wilcoxon rank-sum to test the difference between two sets of normally distributed data. However, the Student t-test is more powerful, and so should be used in preference where the data are normally distributed. The rank-sum test is reserved for skewed data, where the t-test cannot be used.

There is no relationship between standard deviation and interquartile range. Interquartile range is a good way of summarising skewed data where the standard deviation (based on the mean) is not appropriate.

Answer to Question 94

E

The first step of EBM involves converting the need for information into an answerable question. To be answerable a question must be focused and should include each of the following four elements:

• A patient or a problem, defined by specific characteristics that are likely to influence the applicability of the evidence

• An intervention: this might be a diagnostic test, a therapeutic intervention, or information concerning prognosis

• A comparison: in questions about diagnosis this might be with a well-established test; for treatment, it might be with placebo or an alternative treatment

• Outcome measures: it is vital to identify outcome measures that are clinically important, rather than those that are easily measured, e.g. angina, re-infarction and death are more important than thallium scan measurements.

EBM requires explicit use of the best available evidence and its applicability is not restricted to those areas where there is randomised controlled trial evidence.

Answer to Question 95

A

Bias means a flaw in study design that leads to a built-in likelihood that the wrong result may be obtained. It cannot be controlled for at the analysis stage. It can be extremely difficult to design studies without potential bias, particularly when there are complex interactions between exposures under study. Techniques such as restriction and stratification are commonly used to reduce potential for bias.

Answer to Question 96

E

Geographical studies, also called ecological studies, are good at generating hypotheses, but not very helpful in testing them.

Cross-sectional studies, also called prevalence studies, look at the number of cases of a disease at a particular point in time. They are not useful for investigating rare diseases or exposures.

In cohort studies, one group with an exposure of interest is selected and compared over time with another cohort without that exposure. If the control group is well selected, then cohort studies are good for examining the effects of rare exposures, but they are not suited to investigating the cause(s) of a rare disease.

An intervention study cannot be used to look for the cause(s) of a disease.

Answer to Question 97

D

The 95% confidence intervals (95% CI) around a value are the range within which there is a 95% chance that the true value lies. Similarly, the 95% CIs around a difference are the range in which there is a 95% chance that the true difference lies.

If the means of two groups have overlapping 95% CIs, then the two groups are not statistically significantly different. If the 95% CI of the difference between two groups overlaps zero, then the difference between the two groups is not statistically significant.

Statistical and clinical significance should not be confused. A very large study can generate very narrow 95% CIs (or very small p values) for very small differences, which may be of no clinical significance at all. By contrast, a small study may fail to show a statistically significant effect even if the effect is both large and clinically important.

Answer to Question 98

C

Categorical variables are not continuous, e.g. drug/placebo, dead/alive. They should be described as percentages or proportions and compared with a chi-squared test.

Normally distributed continuous data should be described as mean and standard deviation and compared with a Student's t-test.

Skewed continuous data should be described as median and range and compared using a test such as the Wilcoxon rank-sum test or the Mann-Whitney U-test.

Answer to Question 99

E

The null hypothesis is always that there is no difference between groups under study.

A type 1 error occurs when 'the null hypothesis is falsely rejected'. In practice this means that the study claims to find a difference that does not really exist, i.e. the result is just a statistical fluke.

A type 2 error occurs when 'the null hypothesis is falsely accepted'. This means that it is claimed that there is no difference between two groups, when in reality the study is simply too small to detect a difference. This type of error can be avoided by making explicit power calculations before embarking on any study. This will answer the question 'if I am studying an outcome that occurs in (say) 20% of a conventionally treated group and want to show a (say) halving in the rate of this outcome, then how many patients do I need to study?'

Answer to Question 100

D

In this study aspirin reduces the risk of DVT/PE from 2.5% to 1.5%: this is an absolute risk reduction of 1% and a proportional (or relative) risk reduction of 1/2.5 =

40%. The NNT to prevent one DVT/PE is 1/absolute risk reduction = 1/0.01 = 100.

Answer to Question 101

C

Whether or not a clinical trial is ethical is governed by the 'uncertainty principle', the fundamental criterion being that both patient and doctor should be substantially uncertain about the appropriateness of each of the trial treatments for that particular patient. If there are strong preferences for one treatment or another (by either the patient or the doctor), then that patient is ineligible: but if both parties are substantially uncertain, then randomisation is appropriate.

Answer to Question 102

B

Skewed data should always be summarized using the median and range. Standard deviation is based on the mean, which is not appropriate for skewed data.

How do you decide if data are skewed? Plot them out and look at them, or find the median and calculate the mean: if these are more than slightly different, then the data is skewed.

Answer to Question 103

A

The clinical significance of a reported reduction in absolute risk, relative risk or odds ratio is not always obvious. The concept of the number needed to treat (NNT) was devised to make this clearer.

If 9.4% of patients given aspirin after myocardial infarction die, compared with 11.8% of those not given aspirin, then the absolute risk reduction produced by aspirin is 11.8 − 9.4 = 2.4%, the relative risk reduction when taking aspirin is 9.4/11.8 = 0.8 (80%), and the NNT is 1 divided by 0.024 = 42, meaning that 42 patients with myocardial infarction must be treated with aspirin to prevent one death.

Answer to Question 104

E

Absolute risk reduction (or increase) = (Risk in group 1) minus (Risk in group 2), which is 2% in this example.

Relative risk is the difference of outcome in one group compared to another = (Risk in group 1) divided by (Risk in group 2). In this case aspirin reduced relative risk by 20%.

The Number Needed to Treat = 1 divided by (Absolute Risk Reduction), which is 1/0.02 or 50 in this example.

Answer to Question 105

D

Chi-squared tests (and variants thereof) are widely used to compare percentages or proportions of categorical data. From the chi-squared statistic a p value is read off a statistical table to give the degree of significance. Traditionally a p value of less than 0.05, indicating a less than 5% probability that a result has arisen by chance, is taken (arbitrarily) as indicating that chance alone is not responsible for the difference between groups.

Normally distributed data can be compared with a Student's *t*-test (with correction for multiple comparisons when appropriate). Skewed continuous data can be compared with a Wilcoxon rank-sum test or a Mann-Whitney U-test.

Pain Relief and Palliative Care

Answer to Question 106

B, J

The clinical picture suggests she has developed bowel obstruction. A plain abdominal radiograph would be likely to demonstrate this and also help exclude constipation as a cause. Oral medication is not likely to be absorbed because she is vomiting, hence the recommendation that it be given via a syringe driver. Metoclopramide is a prokinetic agent and can make intestinal colic worse: cyclizine is the antiemetic of first choice.

Avoid a nasogastric tube if possible, but it may give symptomatic relief if vomiting is profuse. Hyoscine butylbromide will help abdominal colic but should be given subcutaneously. Carcinoma of the ovary can cause multiple sites of obstruction: surgery is unlikely to be appropriate in this case, and calling a surgeon is not one of the first two things to do.

Answer to Question 107

B, G

Titrating opioids and adding in co-analgesic drugs for neuropathic pain are the manoeuvres most likely to produce initial improvement in her pain. Intrathecal infusions for neuropathic pain should be tried if standard treatment fails. Further oncological management (radio or chemotherapy) is unlikely to benefit the patient in the short term. Topical treatments (fentanyl patch) are best used when pain is stable because of the long dosing intervals. Parenteral approaches (syringe driver) are unlikely to offer better analgesia if the patient is able to absorb oral medicines. Bisphosphonates and paracetamol are appropriate approaches for bone pain rather than neuropathic pain.

Answer to Question 108

A, H

The woman has intestinal obstruction and requires analgesia as opposed to sedation. Diamorphine prn will allow you to calculate how much extra diamorphine needs to be added to the syringe driver. Hyoscine butylbromide is an antispasmodic and will reduce abdominal colic. A nasogastric tube may help, particularly if there is persistent vomiting, but should be avoided if possible. Further investigation of the obstruction would only be appropriate if the patient were fit enough for surgery, and not before an attempt had been made to control symptoms.

Answer to Question 109

D

160 mg oxycodone over 24 hours is equivalent to 320 mg morphine which is equivalent to approx 106 mg diamorphine.

Answer to Question 110

D

Hyoscine, cyclizine and levomepromazine have significant antimuscarinic effects that reduce colonic peristalsis and cause constipation. All 5HT3 antagonists (including ondansetron) cause constipation by inhibiting large bowel transit by blocking cholinergic mechanisms. Haloperidol is a dopamine antagonist and not commonly associated with constipation.

Answer to Question 111

E

Hypercalcaemia may well cause these symptoms and should always be checked unless a patient is clearly dying. Another possible metabolic cause of this presentation is renal failure. Opiates rarely cause confusion in the absence of renal failure or overdose for other reasons.

Answer to Question 112

C

Patients with relapsed ovarian cancer do not infrequently develop renal obstruction due to pelvic recurrence. If they are on morphine they may get accumulation of this drug and signs of opioid toxicity superimposed on the signs of renal failure.

Answer to Question 113

E

The dose of diamorphine should be 1/3 of the total 24-hour dose of morphine. The prn dose should be 1/6 of the 24 hour dose of diamorphine.

Answer to Question 114

D

Fentanyl Conversion Table

Oral 24 hour morphine dose	Fentanyl dose (μg/hr)
Less than 135 mg	25
135–224	50
225–314	75
315–404	100
405–494	125

Emergency Medicine

Answer to Question 115

E

The ECG shows 3rd degree (complete) heart block, with P waves completely dissociated from the QRS complexes. The narrow QRS complexes indicate that the focus for ventricular activity is high in the ventricular conduction system.

Answer to Question 116

A

There is dense consolidation of the right upper lobe, caused in this case by staphylococcal pneumonia following the 'flu.

Answer to Question 117

C, D

Adult basic life support involves:
(1) Check that the situation is safe.
(2) Check responsiveness: shake and shout.
(3) Open airway: head tilt/chin lift.
(4) Check breathing: look/listen.
(5) If breathing: recovery position.
(6) If not breathing: assess circulation: 10 seconds only.
(7) Circulation present: continue rescue breathing.
(8) Circulation not present: compress chest: 100/min, 15:2 ratio.

Answer to Question 118

D

This presentation is typical of Wernicke–Korsakoff syndrome, caused by thiamine deficiency, most often seen in alcoholics, but to be considered in all patients with malnutrition. The features are confusion, ataxia, ophthalmoplegia and nystagmus. The neurological signs do tend to improve with 3 days of parenteral thiamine, but there are often residual memory problems. CT of the head is likely to be normal. An MRI may show evidence of neuronal loss and demyelination in the midbrain structures.

Answer to Question 119

C

Abnormal blood clotting following paracetamol overdose is a good early marker of synthetic liver function. The INR rises first because Factor VII has the shortest half-life, but it is unusual to see any abnormality in blood clotting less than 18 hours from ingestion, so normal INR at 4 hours is unhelpful. An abnormal INR at the time of admission may indicate chronic liver disease, warfarin ingestion or suggest that ingestion of the drug occurred earlier than the patient reports.

Activated charcoal is only likely to be beneficial if given within 1 hour of ingestion of paracetamol.

If the patient complains of tinnitus, this suggests concurrent salicylate consumption, which requires specific treatment according to the plasma level.

Hepatic encephalopathy rarely occurs less than 48 hours from consumption of paracetamol, and reduction in level of consciousness before this is usually a result of concurrent consumption of alcohol, sedative drugs or hypoglycaemia.

Answer to Question 120

C

Thrombolysis probably improves the outcome of patients with large pulmonary emboli (PE) and signs of right heart failure. Thrombolysis removes the clot obstructing the large pulmonary arteries as well as any clot in the pelvic or deep leg veins. It also reduces the release of serotonin and other neurohumoral factors that tend to exacerbate pulmonary hypertension. Contraindications to thrombolysis include recent surgery, trauma and intracranial pathology.

D-dimer is useful as a negative predictor: patients at low risk of PE and with a normal D-dimer level do not require further investigation and can be reassured, but a high D-dimer level is not helpful as a measure of the size of an embolus.

Answer to Question 121

C

Beta blocker overdose may cause dizziness, hypotension, syncope and heart failure. Bradycardia is a common feature of significant overdose and should be treated by the administration of atropine. Intravenous glucagon may also be given, particularly in patients with haemodynamic compromise. Temporary cardiac pacing may be necessary in patients unresponsive to drug therapy.

Answer to Question 122

D

The history clearly suggests anaphylaxis and treatment with intramuscular epinephrine (0.5 ml of 1/1000) is required. In extremis, epinephrine can be given intravenously, but at reduced dosage: make a 1/10 000 solution (by diluting 1 ml of 1/1000 to 10 ml with 0.9% saline) and give this at 1 ml/min (0.1 mg/min) until a response has been obtained (or a total of 0.5 mg—5 ml—has been given).

Answer to Question 123

C

The options to be considered, prior to temporary transvenous pacing, in this context are:

- Atropine 0.5–1.0 mg intravenous bolus, repeated as required.
- Isoprenaline, intravenous infusion at 2–10 μg/min.
- External cardiac pacing.

Answer to Question 124

A

Reactions to *N*-acetyl cysteine (NAC) are well recognised and are not related to hypersensitivity. NAC can almost always be restarted and total dose safely administered after symptomatic treatment. Oral methionine may be an alternative but is definitely second line. IV chlorpromazine would make hypotension worse and should not be given. Withholding treatment and waiting more than 12 hours would expose patient to risk of liver failure.

Infectious Diseases

Answer to Question 125

A

Figure 3 shows suppurative lymphadenitis caused by atypical mycobacterial infection.

The appearance of this problem 4 weeks after starting anti-retroviral treatment is an immune reconstitution phenomenon, when previously subclinical opportunistic infection—commonly TB or CMV—becomes apparent as a result of improvement in immune function.

Anti-retroviral treatment can usually be continued, but sometimes steroids are given to damp down the inflammatory response.

Answer to Question 126

B

The patient has extensive warts caused by papilloma virus. Disease of the extent shown would be most unusual in an immunocompetent host and suggests cell-mediated immunodeficiency.

Papilloma viruses are oncogenic and associated with genital and cutaneous squamous cell carcinomas. There is no specific antiviral therapy: treatment in this case will be by prolonged topical therapy, e.g. podophyllin preparations or cryotherapy, also probably by reduction in immunosuppression dosage.

Answer to Question 127

C

The most likely cause is an amoebic liver abscess, with a pyogenic abscess next on the list of differential diagnoses.

A specific serological test, e.g. immunofluorescent antibody test (IFAT), would be positive in 90% of cases, and cysts may be visible in the stool of 20–30%, but diagnostic/therapeutic aspiration may be needed to exclude pyogenic disease.

Metronidazole is used for acute treatment and diloxanide furoate to eradicate cysts in the bowel lumen.

Answer to Question 128

D

The blood film shows Howell-Jolly bodies, indicating hyposplenism. Patients without a functioning spleen are at particular risk from encapsulated bacteria and pneumococcal sepsis is the most likely diagnosis in this case. His illness could have been prevented by prophylactic penicillin.

Answer to Question 129
E

Figure 7 shows a precipitate of cryoglobulins revealed after blood is taken and kept warm until clotted, centrifuged and the serum removed and stored at 4°C. The cryoprecipitate has settled at the bottom of the tube.

Cryoglobulins are found in some lymphoproliferative disorders, autoimmune diseases and infections, the latter including EBV, hepatitis B and C, and mycoplasma. Hepatitis C causes mixed essential cryoglobulinaemia and can present with the nephrotic syndrome, making this the most likely diagnosis in this case.

Answer to Question 130
E

Figure 8 shows conjunctivitis, most likely due to adenoviral infection in this clinical context.

Herpes simplex can also cause conjunctivitis, and fluorescein instillation is essential to look for ulceration if this is suspected. Possible bacterial causes include *Haemophilus* spp, staphylococci and rarely *Neisseria* spp, but these do not fit well with the clinical scenario in this case.

Answer to Question 131
D

Figure 9 shows Gram-positive rods due to *Clostridium perfringens* causing gas gangrene.

Extensive surgical debridement of all necrotic tissue is essential, along with treatment with high-dose intravenous benzylpenicillin.

Answer to Question 132
C

The patient has had a thoracoplasty where the upper ribs on the left side have been removed to compress the chest cavity to treat pulmonary tuberculosis in the pre-antibiotic era. This was successful in many cases, but often produced a severe kyphoscoliosis, as seen here.

Answer to Question 133
A, B

The differential diagnosis is wide in this context. In this early stage, before a precise diagnosis has been made, he needs good broad-spectrum antibiotics aimed at covering immediate life-threatening infections such as meningo-coccal, pneumococcal or gram-negative sepsis. Drug, mode of delivery and dosing should allow adequate CSF penetration in the event that he has meningitis. Given his age and predisposing haematological condition listeria must be considered, hence ampicillin should be given in addition to a broad-spectrum agent such as ceftriaxone. The addition of aciclovir whilst awaiting PCR on CSF is not inappropriate but this should be administered intravenously.

Answer to Question 134
C, D

This would be a typical picture of a Gram negative or *Staphylococcus aureus* bacteraemia complicating surgical instrumentation. Often there is no immediate febrile response. The antibiotic regimen selected should have good Gram-negative cover and also activity against MRSA given his screening result. Other causes of acute post-operative deterioration, e.g. myocardial infarction, must be excluded and standard resuscitation performed.

Answer to Question 135
C, I

This woman has several pointers to potentially severe malarial disease – she is drowsy, jaundiced and pregnant.

Even when patients have severe cerebral malaria, CT seldom adds anything to diagnosis, and jaundice is common in malaria due to red-cell breakdown. Low platelets are almost invariable in this condition and require no treatment unless a patient is bleeding. Prophylactic antibiotics and phenobarbitone are seldom helpful, even in severe cases. Steroids are actively unhelpful. Exchange transfusion should only be contemplated in those with very high peripheral parasite loads (10% would be a minimum, usually more – always ask for specialist advice).

The key to managing malaria is an appropriate anti-malarial given early, and this takes priority over all else. In potentially severe cases this should always be parenteral and as she has low platelets, intravenous is preferable to intramuscular. Hypoglycaemia is a common complication in severe malaria, especially in pregnant women, and those who are drowsy should have their glucose measured repeatedly.

Answer to Question 136
C, J

British Thoracic Society guidelines for the treatment of severe community-acquired pneumonia suggest parenteral treatment with a second- or third-generation cephalosporin, with high dose parenteral erythromycin in suspected Legionnaire's disease, which proved to be the diagnosis in this case.

Answer to Question 137

A

Other than rickettsial infection, which usually presents with a localised lymphadenopathy +/− eschar and rash and normal white blood count, all the other conditions listed can be associated with peripheral neutrophilia. Malaria is rarely associated with raised neutrophils but should always be excluded in travellers returning from endemic areas. Amoebic liver abscess is associated with neutrophilia and not eosinophilia. Always remember that many travellers with fever will have cosmopolitan rather than exotic causes for their illness, but a careful history and examination should be undertaken to exclude the exotic causes.

Answer to Question 138

C

Schistosomiasis is not endemic in the Indian subcontinent, although it would be a cause of this presentation elsewhere in the tropics. Heavy worm loads with *Trichuris* can cause bloody diarrhoea. Cosmopolitan causes of bloody diarrhoea should always be considered as a cause despite the travel history and *C. difficile* disease excluded when antibiotics have been taken.

Answer to Question 139

D

This is the typical presentation of someone with dengue fever, which has an incubation period of 5 to 8 days. Both malaria (usually falciparum in Thailand) and typhoid would have to be excluded. The diagnosis of dengue is confirmed serologically.

Dermatology

Answer to Question 140

C

The appearances are those of guttate psoriasis. This is often triggered by a streptococcal throat infection and presents as an acute shower of small (<1 cm) plaques ('rain drops') over the trunk and limbs.

Guttate psoriasis can be confused with pityriasis rosea or secondary syphilis, but the clinical context in this case is typical of guttate psoriasis.

Answer to Question 141

D

This is allergic contact dermatitis to nickel, caused in this typical case by contact with the stud fastener of a pair of jeans.

Answer to Question 142

E

The V-shaped cut off at the neck is absolutely typical of a photo-induced rash. The patient had been prescribed a thiazide diuretic in the autumn, but the rash did not appear until the following spring when he began spending time outdoors gardening.

Answer to Question 143

B, F

Oral and genital ulceration may be part of Behçet's disease, for which a pathergy test is helpful, but cutaneous ulcers makes this diagnosis unlikely. Skin scrapings, which are generally sent for mycology and thus for diagnosis of fungal infections, would not be helpful. The history is not suggestive of an allergic contact dermatitis or atopic dermatitis so investigations such as patch tests, skin prick tests and IgE levels would not be helpful.

Ulceration of the skin, genitalia and mouth can occur in autoimmune blistering diseases such as pemphigus vulgaris (PV). The patient is the right age and ethnic group for PV that tends to present more commonly in the 3rd–6th decades and in Jewish and Indian patients. A skin biopsy for routine histology is a useful investigation, but the gold standard is direct immunofluorescence (performed on a skin biopsy), which demonstrates the intercellular IgG in the epidermis, which characterises PV.

Answer to Question 144

D, F

A precipitant is identified in about 50% of patients with chronic urticaria, but IgE-mediated chronic urticaria is a relatively minor cause. It is not associated with internal malignancy, but can rarely be associated with systemic vasculitides although in the vast majority of cases there are no vasculitic changes on biopsy. H1-antagonists can be very helpful and H2-antagonists can help some patients. Most patients with chronic urticaria will have improved within a year, but relapses are not infrequent. For uncomplicated chronic urticaria with no clear clues from the history or examination of systemic disease or an exogenous precipitant, the current UK guidelines (2003) recommend full blood count, ESR and antinuclear antibodies as reasonable screening investigations for those with moderate-severe disease. Non-steroidals are a common cause of exacerbation of urticaria.

Answer to Question 145

E

Rheumatoid arthritis is a risk factor for pyoderma gangrenosum (PG). The anterior shin is an unusual site for venous ulceration and Dopplers are normal, making arterial disease unlikely. PG ulcers are often painful and do not respond to conventional treatment.

PG is associated with pathergy, such that trauma to the ulcer via debridement, or removal of skin at a distant site for grafting, would be contraindicated. PG is diagnosed by exclusion of other causes of ulceration and by its improvement with immunosuppression.

Answer to Question 146

A

The two most common causes of scarring alopecia are lichen planopilaris (lichen planus affecting the scalp hair follicles) and discoid lupus erythematosus. Both conditions cause inflammation and can be difficult to differentiate clinically.

Androgenetic alopecia and alopecia areata are both non-scarring causes of alopecia. Traction alopecia can cause scarring but is not usually associated with inflammation: it occurs at sites of traction and is usually caused by hair styling practices, such as braiding.

Haematology

Answer to Question 147

B

The blood film shows macrocytosis, poikilocytosis, oval macrocytes and hypersegmented neutrophils, all characteristic of B12 deficiency (pernicious anaemia).

Answer to Question 148

C

There are blast cells with nucleoli and granules. There is no myeloid differentiation, which would be expected in chronic myeloid leukaemia, and the white cell count is not very high. There are no plasma cells or lymphocytes seen on the film.

Answer to Question 149

D

The obvious suspicion is of a thrombosis of the left axillary or subclavian vein, and the correct investigative technique is venography to demonstrate this. Blood D-dimers should not be requested when there is a high clinical probability of venous thromboembolic disease, as is clearly the case here. A normal D-dimer is very useful in excluding venous thromboembolic disease when there is a low index of clinical suspicion.

Answer to Question 150

E

The blood film shows clumping of red cells caused by cold agglutinins typical of mycoplasma infection. This clumping has led to false elevation of the mean corpuscular volume as estimated by the automated Coulter counter.

Answer to Question 151

E

The blood film shows mature lymphocytes typical of chronic lymphatic leukaemia (CLL), cell markers confirming that they were CD5 and CD19 positive. CLL is often picked up as an incidental finding.

Answer to Question 152

B, E

Immune mediated thrombocytopenia (ITP) is an immunological disorder characterised by premature platelet destruction due to production of antibodies directed against platelet antigens. Destruction is mediated by the spleen and liver. Treatment options in a bleeding patient at presentation are corticosteroids, e.g. prednisolone at a dose of 1 mg/kg body weight. Intravenous immunoglobulins can be used to bring about a rapid rise in the platelet count, but its effect is not long-lasting. It works by blocking the Fc receptor on macrophages and preventing phagocytosis. Platelet infusions can be given for life threatening bleeds, but a substantial number of units (not a single unit) will be needed to swamp the antibody. Chemotherapeutic agents such as vincristine, cyclophosphamide and even combination chemotherapy have been tried in refractory cases. FFP and/or leucocyte infusions have no role in the management of ITP, and heparin can exacerbate the bleeding diathesis.

Answer to Question 153

F, H

Von Willebrand's disease occurs in 1% of the population and could present in this way. Acquired bleeding problems such as DIC, liver disease, ITP or uraemia are excluded by the length of the history. Von Willebrand's factor (VWF) is the carrier for factor VIII and in Von Willebrand's disease the activated prothrombin time (APTT) may be prolonged due to a low factor VIII level. Specific assays include those for VWF and ristocetin cofactor. Treatment in this case might include oral iron (to correct iron deficiency) and the use of DDAVP (which promotes release of VWF) intranasally at the time of the menses to reduce blood loss. Operative procedures can be covered with intravenous DDAVP. Do not forget to take a family history: others may be affected (autosomal dominant).

Answer to Question 154

C, H

Splenectomy is not without hazard. It is reserved for symptomatic anaemia that affects quality of life. Vaccination and lifelong penicillin are required in adults. Splenectomy removes the source of red cell destruction and spherocytes may rise in number on the blood film. Splenectomy is performed in older rather than young children, but is not routine.

Answer to Question 155

B, E

Although it is important to seek help from senior colleagues, you should be able to make a decision on this. Don't leave this sort of problem to a later date or to somebody else: if the patient is lost to follow up they could become quite ill. The blood film will show if there is polychromasia (immune haemolysis) or features of megaloblastic anaemia. The film will give you more information than just a reticulocyte count (is this high in megaloblastic anaemia?). The B12 and folate levels should be checked quickly because restoring these haematinics can make people feel a lot better very quickly.

Answer to Question 156

C, I

The father's blood group is not relevant (and paternity cannot always be assumed). The ABO blood group is also not relevant. Anti D is used when the mother is RhD-ve and the child RhD+ve.

Answer to Question 157

A, E

Although all of the causes listed can result in a transfusion reaction (of varying severity), the most common reason for a severe reaction to blood is transfusion of the incorrect unit. In almost all cases this is due to human error, from incorrect labelling of blood samples to failing to check the details on the unit being given. Best practice is that addressograph labels should not be allowed on the sample bottle and forms and sample bottle must be signed by the person performing the venepuncture.

Answer to Question 158

B, E

Both malaria and HIV infection (and AIDS) classically present with a low lymphocyte count. All the other conditions listed would tend to be associated with a lymphocytosis.

Answer to Question 159

D

The good prognostic features in childhood ALL are age between one and 10 yrs, female gender, low white cell count (below 50×10^9/l), no evidence of central nervous system disease or particular chromosomal abnormalities and complete response to early chemotherapy. Haemoglobin concentration and platelet count do not significantly influence prognosis.

Answer to Question 160

B

The clue is the raised reticulocyte count, which causes the raised mean corpuscular volume (MCV). This is due to Coombs' positive haemolysis – seen in 10% of cases of chronic lymphocytic leukaemia (CLL). Although B12, folate and iron deficiency can occur in CLL, they do not raise the reticulocyte count. A marrow aspirate would not give the answer here.

Answer to Question 161

D

Most patients with Waldenström's or myeloma relapse with a rise in their paraprotein. When measured, this man's IgM had risen to 29 g/l and his anaemia was due to active disease. He developed chest pain due to an acute haemolytic transfusion reaction that caused the Coombs' test to become positive. This was due to a Jka red cell antibody that had not previously been detected.

The plasma viscosity is only slightly raised and is unlikely to produce renal failure at this level. Fludarabine can cause Coombs' positive haemolysis, but not usually 5 years after treatment. There is no evidence for acute myeloid leukaemia (AML).

Answer to Question 162

C

Bone pain is a common presenting feature of multiple myeloma. In 80% of patients with myeloma there is a paraprotein in the serum, usually of the IgG or IgA class. However, in 20% of patients only free light chains are produced (Bence-Jones only myeloma). Stick tests of the urine do not detect Bence-Jones proteins.

Answer to Question 163

D

The British Committee for Standards in Haematology (BCSH) has published guidelines for reversal of warfarin effect. A patient who is not bleeding and who has no additional risk factors for bleeding (e.g. older age, peptic ulceration etc), with an INR less than 8 may stop their warfarin and wait for the level to come down without intervention.

Oncology

Answer to Question 164

C

There are multiple hot spots in the axial skeleton due to bone metastases and a non-functioning left kidney due to long-standing obstruction.

Answer to Question 165

B

There is post-radiation fibrosis of the right upper lobe: note the geometrically delineated shadowing that corresponds to the radiation field and tracheal and mediastinal shift due to contraction of the irradiated lung.

Answer to Question 166

F, G

Squamous carcinomas rarely cause brain metastases. Melanoma is the most common primary site after lung cancer and breast cancer.

Answer to Question 167

D, I

For most patients who present with metastatic disease, routine examination and investigation will rapidly disclose the underlying primary tumour. However, for 1–5% the primary site remains obscure because it is too small to be detected or has regressed.

Women with isolated axillary lymphadenopathy (adenocarcinoma or undifferentiated carcinoma) should be managed as stage II breast cancer and have a similar prognosis (65% 5-year survival). Women with peritoneal carcinomatosis (often papillary carcinoma with elevated serum CA-125) should be managed as stage III ovarian cancer.

Answer to Question 168

D, E

Cardiac manifestations occur in 11% to 66% of patients with carcinoid syndrome, typically fibrosis of the endocardium of the right side of the heart, although left side lesions can also occur. The fibrous deposits are diffuse and most commonly affect the ventricular aspect of the tricuspid valve and associated chordae, less commonly the pulmonary valve cusps. They cause constriction of both the tricuspid and pulmonary valves: stenosis is usually the predominant effect at the pulmonary valve, whereas at the tricuspid valve the constriction results in the valve being fixed open and regurgitation is usually predominant.

Answer to Question 169

A

You should have a high index of suspicion about spinal cord compression which needs to be diagnosed and treated as an emergency in order to have the best possible outcome. Underlying infections are common in this elderly and debilitated group and should be considered, particularly if there is non-specific deterioration.

Answer to Question 170

D

The first priority should be resection of the sigmoid lesion to prevent large bowel obstruction. Two liver lesions confined to the same lobe may be suitable for liver resection, with chemotherapy either before or after resection.

Answer to Question 171

A

Osteoid osteoma is a benign bone tumour with a central small nidus of osteoid that incites a vigorous reaction in surrounding tissue. It is characteristically found in the femur, tibia, talus, spine and humerus, usually in the diaphysis or metaphysis of these bones. The most common presentation is with pain unrelated to activity, sometimes exacerbated by drinking alcohol, and often be relieved by non-steroidal anti-inflammatory drugs. Osteoid osteomas are most common in males (M:F, 3:1) between 7 and 25 years of age.

Answer to Question 172

E

Although metastatic breast cancer can present in countless ways, the possibility of a second malignancy should be considered – in this case possibly an operable lung cancer. If the pattern of recurrence is characteristic, for example multiple bone or liver metastases, then a confirmatory biopsy is not generally required.

Answer to Question 173

A

The standard treatment of early breast cancer is wide local excision and axillary node sampling followed by adjuvant breast radiotherapy. This achieves similar local control and survival rates to mastectomy with less mutilating surgery.

Women without axillary node involvement can be divided into a high risk group (tumour >1 cm or does not express the Estrogen Receptor, ER), who should be given adjuvant treatment, and a low risk group (smaller ER-positive) who do not require adjuvant treatment. Women with histological spread to axillary nodes should receive adjuvant chemotherapy, which delays recurrence and improves survival.

Cardiology

Answer to Question 174

C

The most likely explanation for the history and physical findings is aortic dissection causing aortic regurgitation and with leakage of blood into the pericardium. The chest radiograph (Figure 21) is not diagnostic, but shows a suspicion of a widened mediastinum that would support this diagnosis. Urgent CT scan of the chest or transoesophageal echocardiography is required to make the diagnosis.

Answer to Question 175

E

The patient had severe mitral regurgitation and the radiograph (Figure 22) shows cardiomegaly with an enlarged left atrium and pulmonary oedema.

Answer to Question 176

E, I

Restoration of sinus rhythm can be achieved pharmacologically or by DC cardioversion. However, DC cardioversion is not likely to lead to permanent restoration of sinus rhythm in a patient who has had previous episodes of AF, hence in this case an attempt at 'chemical cardioversion' is appropriate. Class III agents – potassium channel blockers that prolong myocyte repolarisation – are most appropriate: sotalol or amiodarone. Digoxin can be used for rate control but does not promote return of sinus rhythm, indeed it's use may make this more unlikely. Class I agents – e.g. quinidine, procaineamide and disopyramide, which prolong the action potential – have been used to try to restore sinus rhythm, but NOT in patients with ischaemic heart disease (such as this man).

Answer to Question 177

C, F

Whenever you approach a patient with a broad complex tachycardia it is always safest to presume they have ventricular tachycardia until proven otherwise. In fact, it is most likely that they will have a ventricular tachycardia rather than one of the other possibilities above, which may produce similar traces on a Holter monitor. Patients with ventricular tachycardia are not always syncopal, indeed right ventricular outflow tract tachycardia usually presents with just palpitations. It occurs as a result of a triggered focus in the right ventricular outflow tract and generally carries an excellent prognosis. It is best treated with radiofrequency ablation. This is in contrast to ischaemic ventricular tachycardia which carries a very poor prognosis unless treated appropriately. In the context of impaired left ventricular function this invariably means with an implantable cardioverter defibrillator (ICD).

Answer to Question 178

E

The guidelines on basic life support identify the importance of early access to defibrillation in cardiac arrest. They therefore suggest that no CPR is commenced until a call for emergency services has been made and the potential for early defibrillation is made possible. Once CPR begins the ratio of compressions to ventilations is 15 to 2. A precordial thump is not indicated in the unwitnessed collapse.

Answer to Question 179
D

This man has ischaemic cardiomyopathy, but no evidence of reversible ischaemia on functional (thallium) assessment. He has had symptomatic VT and therefore is at high risk of sudden death. Current evidence suggests that he will gain prognostic benefit from implantation of an implantable cardioverter defibrillator. Beta-blockers have also been shown to independently improve prognosis (and symptoms) in patients with impaired left ventricular function.

Answer to Question 180
B

Pacemaker types are identified by a 3 or 4 letter code. The first letter indicates the chamber paced (A = atrium; V = ventricle; D = both or dual), the second letter represents which chamber is sensed; and the third is what response the pacemaker gives to a sensed beat (I = inhibit; T = trigger; D = both). The fourth, usually R (rate responsive) is for more sophisticated technologies. In this case of complete heart block, in order to maintain AV synchrony, a dual chamber pacemaker is required (DDD). Assuming the atrial (p wave) rate is normal the function will be generally sensing the p wave and then pacing the ventricle.

Answer to Question 181
B

This man has severe aortic stenosis and concomitant coronary artery disease. Whilst it is impossible to differentiate which lesion is causing his current symptoms, symptomatic aortic stenosis is associated with significantly impaired prognosis and surgical intervention is warranted. Percutaneous aortic valvotomy is relatively unsuccessful in adults, with rapid restenosis.

Answer to Question 182
D

Clinically this man has an infected mitral valve replacement with a severe paravalvular leak. Following surgery the commonest infecting organisms (up to around 9 months) are coagulase negative staphylococci. Antibiotics alone will not cure the infection; the valve must be

replaced again. In this case this should be with a metallic valve since a bioprosthetic valve would be likely to need replacing after 10–15 years due to degeneration, thereby subjecting him to a high-risk third operation. Bioprosthetic and metallic valves have similar risk for subsequent endocarditis.

Answer to Question 183
D

Given the lack of signs and family history of sudden death the most likely diagnosis is pulmonary hypertension. Further investigations would include transthoracic echocardiography and left and right cardiac catheterisation.

Respiratory Medicine

Answer to Question 184
C

There is right-sided pneumothorax.

Answer to Question 185
A

The chest radiograph (Figure 24) shows bilateral alveolar shadowing due to amiodarone-induced interstitial lung disease. Pulmonary oedema could cause identical radiographic appearances in the lungs, but the normal heart sounds (no gallop rhythm) and normal sized heart on the radiograph are both against this diagnosis.

Answer to Question 186
C, J

The most common cause of haemoptysis in a young patient is pulmonary infection, either with pyogenic bacteria or mycobacterium tuberculosis depending on the clinical context. The short history with previous good health makes TB unlikely in this case. A clear chest examination is not unusual in pneumonia, particularly in the context of atypical or viral pathogens. The next most common causes would be bronchiectasis (made unlikely in this case by the absence of any previous respiratory problems) or pulmonary embolism. Tumour (benign or malignant), Goodpasture's syndrome or pulmonary vasculitis (often as part of a pulmonary-renal syndrome) also need to be considered but are much less likely diagnoses.

Answer to Question 187

A, B

Near fatal asthma or brittle asthma is responsible for around 1000 deaths every year in the UK. It mainly occurs in young patients, previous attacks and a short time between the start of symptoms and hospital admission being the two main risk factors. The treatment of choice is hospitalisation with early start of nebulised bronchodilators, oxygen and intravenous corticosteroids. The recovery rate is normally quick. Long acting beta-2 agonists and leukotrine receptor antagonists are not successful in preventing near fatal asthma. There is no relationship between near fatal asthma and personal history of allergy. The incidence of the disease does not differ according to gender and there are no seasonal variations for the rate of hospitalisation.

Answer to Question 188

C

This patient is in Step Two of asthma treatment, but his asthma is not well controlled as he needs to take his rescue medication more than twice a day. His treatment should be stepped up. In Step Three of asthma treatment, guidelines from the British Thoracic Society advise first adding inhaled long-acting beta-2 agonist (LABA) and then re-assessing the situation. If there is a good response to LABA, this medication should be continued. If there is benefit from LABA but control is still inadequate, LABA should be continued, and the inhaled corticosteroids should be increased to a high dose. If there is no response to LABA, then that treatment should be stopped and inhaled corticosteroids should be increased to a high dose.

Answer to Question 189

A

Resuscitation is the first priority. Maximum inspired oxygen should be given by facemask: this is best achieved using a reservoir bag at a flow rate of 15 l/min, which can generate an FiO_2 of about 85%. Nebulised salbutamol (5–10 mg) driven by oxygen should be given, and many would add ipatropium bromide (Atrovent, 500 μg) to the nebuliser chamber at the same time as the salbutamol. If the woman does not improve, then call for assistance from the Intensive Care Unit (ICU) sooner rather than later. Although it is always important to consider pneumothorax in any breathless patient, there is no evidence at all to suggest that this woman has bilateral pneu-

mothoraces and she would not be well served by chest decompression.

Answer to Question 190

D

Long-term oxygen treatment is recommended if pO_2 is less than 7.3 kPa on two occasions in remission of COPD. This patient's pO_2 is likely to improve when he recovers from his current exacerbation and his ABG should be rechecked in about 6 weeks time. As he seems able to tolerate his mild hypoxia, he would not require any oxygen supplementation at home at this stage.

Answer to Question 191

D

Steroid challenge is indicated in chronic obstructive pulmonary disease (COPD) of more than moderate severity. Standard practice would be to give prednisolone 30 mg daily for 2 weeks, regarding an increase in FEV1 of >10% and >200 ml as a positive response. Given the non-specific effects and many side effects of steroids, it is crucial to demonstrate functional improvement: many patients with COPD have sustained severe complications of steroid treatment, e.g. vertebral fracture, without any evidence that the steroids were beneficial for their chest.

Answer to Question 192

A

The history strongly suggests pneumonia 6 weeks previously that has failed to clear. Empyema could cause persistent fever, malaise and breathlessness, but would not explain continued sputum production. Alcoholism is a risk factor for aspiration and cavitating pneumonia. Bronchiectasis typically causes chronic breathlessness and sputum production, often with febrile infective exacerbations, but will not be the diagnosis in a patient with a short respiratory history.

Answer to Question 193

E

Although all of the diagnoses listed could present in this way, pneumonia with effusion/empyema is much the most likely. Examination of the pleural fluid is critical. If associated with pneumonia and the effusion is opaque/turbid and smells foul then it is clearly an empyema, which would also be suggested by pH < 7.2.

Gastroenterology and Hepatology

Answer to Question 194

A

The radiograph (Figure 25) shows a very dilated colon (toxic megacolon), which is a medical emergency. Aside from resuscitation and supportive care she requires intravenous antimicrobials, intravenous steroids and immediate liaison with surgical services familiar with this problem – emergency colectomy may be required.

Answer to Question 195

D

The barium enema (Figure 26) shows a classic 'apple core' lesion just proximal to the splenic flexure, which is due to a colonic carcinoma.

Answer to Question 196

E, H

Combination therapy with alpha-interferon (which may be pegylated in order to produce smoother drug level profiles and reduce side effects) and ribavirin is now considered standard therapy of chronic hepatitis C infection. The development of new anti-virals and new combinations of existing anti-virals offer hope for the future but currently have no place outside of clinical trials.

Answer to Question 197

C, J

Fluid resuscitation can be carried out via multiple large bore peripheral lines. Subclavian line placement can be hazardous and is contra-indicated in patients with coagulopathy, the internal jugular vein being the location of choice if central venous monitoring is required. Not all patients will experience alcohol withdrawal and benzodiazepines should be avoided if possible in patients who are encephalopathic. Sequestration of platelets in a spleen enlarged as a result of portal hypertension is the usual cause of thrombocytopaenia in this scenario. Therapeutic paracentesis should only be considered if ascites is tense, but diagnostic paracentesis should be carried out, covered with antibiotics in this case in view of the GI bleed. A number of studies have shown that somatostatin analogues are as effective in controlling acute variceal haemorrhage as interventional endoscopy, and drugs should be commenced while waiting for endoscopy. Although TIPSS was initially considered 'a bridge to transplantation', it may be used in patients with uncontrollable portal hypertensive haemorrhage, although deterioration in encephalopathy may result. In patients with cirrhosis at least 60% of gastrointestinal haemorrhage will be due to varices. Oesophageal banding is now the accepted intervention for bleeding oesophageal varices, but sclerotherapy is an accepted alternative where local experience of banding does not exist. Beta-blockade has been shown to be effective in secondary prophylaxis of variceal haemorrhage.

Answer to Question 198

D

An isolated hyperbilirubinaemia is invariably due to Gilbert's syndrome (4% of the population) and should be regarded as a variant of normal. The most important condition in adulthood that could give similar liver function test results would be haemolytic anaemia: a reticulocyte count (raised) and serum haptoglobin (low) would differentiate.

Answer to Question 199

C

At the time of clinical acute hepatitis B with onset of jaundice, there is active viral replication with elevated HBV DNA levels and presence of e antigen and surface antigen. High serum transaminase levels are common, although a cholestatic phase with high alkaline phosphatase levels can occur following the transaminitis in 5%. Subsequently e antibodies develop, followed by surface antibodies in most individuals who clear the virus. Evidence of previous infection is indicated by the presence of antibodies to core protein and surface protein. Those individuals who have been immunised will have antibodies to the surface protein only.

Answer to Question 200

C

This woman has cholangitis, which complicates common bile duct (CBD) stones but not biliary malignancy unless a biliary stent has previously been inserted and has blocked. Primary sclerosing cholangitis can be complicated by cholangitis but this would be unusual. Do not forget that elderly patients rarely complain of pain and that common bile duct stones may be present several years after a cholecystectomy. About 75% of CBD stones can be delineated by ultrasound, although detection is less likely if the bile ducts are not dilated.

Answer to Question 201

A

Chronic hepatitis C is a very common cause of minor elevations in serum transaminases. Other liver function tests can be entirely normal and assessment of viral status by PCR along with histological assessment may be needed, particularly if treatment is being considered. Isolated elevations in AST (aspartate aminotransferase) can occur with muscle disease and the AST:ALT ratio can be useful in diagnosing alcoholic liver disease, because more than two-thirds of patients will have a ratio greater than 2. Menstruating women are generally protected against haemochromatosis. Wilson's disease is rare but must always be considered in a young person with chronic hepatitis.

Answer to Question 202

C

This patient has evidence of chronic liver disease with portal hypertension, hence a diagnosis of bleeding oesophageal varices is most likely. Intravenous terlipressin reduces variceal pressure following bleeding and may influence prognosis. Propranolol is beneficial in primary and secondary prevention of variceal haemorrhage in the long term, but has no role in the acute setting. Intravenous proton pump inhibitors may be beneficial in patients with actively bleeding peptic ulceration, but have no role in variceal bleeding. Intravenous ranitidine has never been shown to affect outcome following gastrointestinal bleeding of any type, while eradication of helicobacter will only be important in the short term if he is shown at endoscopy to have peptic ulceration as a cause for his bleeding.

Answer to Question 203

D

Hepatic steatosis is associated with diabetes mellitus, hypercholesterolaemia, hypertriglyceridaemia and obesity. Diagnosis may require liver biopsy, although resolution of abnormal liver blood test results on correction of hyperglycaemia, hyperlipidaemia or obesity may make this unnecessary.

Answer to Question 204

C

Until recently interferon was the first-line treatment for chronic hepatitis B infection associated with elevated serum transaminases. However, this is contraindicated in the presence of end-stage liver disease (cirrhosis with elevated bilirubin and prothrombin time in this case) because it can lead to liver failure. Lamivudine suppresses HBV replication and is safe to use in decompensated end-stage cirrhosis.

Ribavirin has no effect on hepatitis B replication but used in combination with interferon is more effective than ribavirin alone in eradicating chronic infection with hepatitis C.

Answer to Question 205

B

Once diuretic resistant ascites has occurred, blood flow to the kidney is reduced and it is easy to precipitate hepatorenal failure. NSAIDs do this by further reducing renal blood flow and should be avoided.

Paracetamol is safe in a dose not exceeding 4 grams/day. Rifampicin can cause cholestasis when used alone but is a useful drug for treating pruritus in biliary diseases when cholestyramine does not work: it can be used in patients with end-stage liver disease providing liver biochemistry is monitored. Although chlordiazepoxide may accumulate, causing encephalopathy, alcoholic withdrawal must be treated/prevented in a cirrhotic who is actively drinking on admission; doses must be titrated on a day-to-day basis.

Answer to Question 206

C

The blood count shows a normocytic anaemia, consistent with the anaemia of chronic disorders and not suggestive of iron deficiency. Acute loss of blood does not lead to any immediate change in the full blood count: haemodilution takes some time to occur, hence the full blood count can never be used to decide whether or not someone has suffered a significant acute haemorrhage. Physical examination will tell you this, the two most reliable signs of intravascular volume depletion being postural hypotension (lying and sitting) and a reduced jugular venous pressure.

Answer to Question 207

B

The Rockall score is often used to assess severity of gastrointestinal haemorrhage and / or to triage patients for emergency endoscopy. Four parameters are used to calculate the Rockall score:
(a) Age (yrs)—< 60 (score 0), 60–79 (1), > 80 (2)
(b) Systolic BP (mmHg) and Pulse (/min)—SBP > 100 with P < 100 (0), SBP > 100 with P > 100 (1), SBP < 100 (2).

(c) Comorbidity—None (0), Other (1), Cardiac failure / ischaemic heart disease (2), renal or liver failure (3).

The total score predicts mortality as follows: Score 0, 0.2%; score 2, 5%; score 4, 24%; score 6, 49%.

Answer to Question 208

C

Helicobacter pylori is associated with 95% of duodenal ulcers and 80% of gastric ulcers. Tests for *H pylori* include serology, histological biopsy, urease testing, urea breath testing and faecal antigen assays. False negative urease testing can occur if patients have been treated with antibiotics, bismuth or proton pump inhibitors in the prior 1–2 weeks. In this case, where a *H pylori*-associated gastritis and duodenal ulcer is most likely, eradication should be prescribed regardless of the urease test.

Neurology

Answer to Question 209

A

The right eye is 'down and out' with a dilated pupil, characteristic of a right third nerve palsy. On attempted down gaze the right eye would rotate inwards, and on attempted gaze to the left the right eye would not move.

Answer to Question 210

C

The CT scan (Figure 28) shows low density lesions in the left hemisphere, with swelling of the left hemisphere causing some midline shift and compression of the left lateral ventricle: this, together with the clinical history, would be consistent with left middle cerebral artery infarction.

Answer to Question 211

D, G

Common presentations of a parietal lobe tumour include contralateral sensory loss, neglect, apraxia and contralateral homonymous field defect, which sometimes consist solely of lower quadrantanopia.

Answer to Question 212

E, G

Tension-type headache is characterized by a constant, non-pulsatile, band-like, bi-fronto-temporal pressure on top of the head. The headache is not worsened by physical activity and can be associated with mild nausea, but not with vomiting. Chronic forms are worsened by anxiety and stress. Alcohol may relieve the headache. Regular simple analgesia may be the commonest cause of chronic daily headache. There are no abnormal features on examination. Amitriptyline is the drug treatment of choice.

Answer to Question 213

E

This man is describing sleep paralysis. Sleep paralysis may be isolated or occur in the context of narcolepsy, affecting 15–45% of patients with this condition. The symptoms represent the atonia of REM sleep. Awareness is preserved during the attack. Although the respiratory muscles are only ever mildly affected in comparison to the limbs, patients may describe a feeling of suffocation that can be particularly frightening.

Answer to Question 214

E

The lateral gaze centre is situated in the pons. A lesion in the right side of the pons will cause impaired conjugate gaze to the right side, with consequent deviation of the eyes to the left. A lesion in the right frontal lobe could cause a left hemiparesis, but if the eyes were affected then they would be directed to the right side and the patient would be unable to look to the left.

Answer to Question 215

C

The left-sided weakness is due to right cerebral hemisphere dysfunction, which with sudden onset is likely to represent a transient ischaemic attack. The combination of this symptom with amaurosis strongly suggests a right internal carotid artery stenosis in this case. Cardioembolism is unlikely in the absence of either atrial fibrillation or previous cardiac symptoms. Transient occlusion of a small penetrating vessel, i.e. a lacunar syndrome, could cause hemiparesis but not amaurosis fugax. Giant cell arteritis should always be considered in patients over 60-years-old, but there are no specific features to support the diagnosis, although it is always worthwhile checking the erythrocyte sedimentation rate (ESR). Migraine equivalents (aura-like symptoms without headache) can provide diagnostic difficulties but there is no suggestion of the characteristic slow spread of symptoms in this patient.

Answer to Question 216

A

The history suggests the dysarthria-clumsy hand syndrome, one of the classic lacunar syndromes that are strokes in the subcortical regions (or brain stem) secondary to small vessel disease. The usual site of damage in the dysarthria-clumsy hand syndrome is the internal capsule or pons, infarction being more common than haemorrhage, although both are caused by disease of small perforating arterioles. Contributory risk factors include smoking, hypertension and hypercholesterolaemia.

Migraine equivalents (aura-like symptoms without headache) can provide diagnostic difficulties and should always be considered in those with a previous history of migraine, but there is no suggestion of the characteristic slow spread of symptoms in this patient.

The neck tongue syndrome consists of pain and parasthesias in one half of the tongue precipitated by neck movement, often associated with occipital pain and ipsilateral hand parasthesias.

Answer to Question 217

B

The diagnosis is internal carotid artery dissection causing a left Horner's syndrome.

Answer to Question 218

A

The investigation of choice in suspected subarachnoid haemorrhage (SAH) is immediate CT scan without contrast, taking very thin cuts through the base of the brain to optimise the chances of seeing small collections of blood. Imaging within 12 hours using modern scanners has a 98–100% sensitivity for SAH. Lumbar puncture should be performed in suspected SAH if the CT scan is not diagnostic. The CSF specimen should be centrifuged without delay and examined by spectrophotometry for the presence of xanthochromia due to the presence of oxyhaemoglobin and bilirubin. Note, however, that xanthochromia may not be present if the CSF is examined within 12 hours of haemorrhage occurring, so lumbar puncture should be delayed for 24 hours.

Answer to Question 219

E

The triad of dementia, urinary incontinence and gait disturbance suggests normal pressure hydrocephalus until proved otherwise.

Answer to Question 220

C

There is some overlap between the different types of dementia, but in this case there are clues that this is dementia with Lewy bodies (DLB) with the early development of instability, falls and hallucinations. Other features include fluctuating cognition, depression and delusions. Treatment is usually symptomatic, but remember that neuroleptic drugs such as haloperidol will worsen Parkinsonian features, so consider using atypical antipsychotic agents such as quetiapine. There is some evidence that the dementia may respond to anticholinesterase inhibitors. Dementia associated with Parkinson's disease tends to occur late in the course of the disease.

Answer to Question 221

C

The combination of progressive cognitive decline, fluctuating symptoms, visual hallucinations, extrapyramidal signs (rigidity and bradykinesia more prominent than tremor) and sleep pattern reversal suggest a diagnosis of Lewy body dementia.

Answer to Question 222

E

The diagnosis is temporal lobe epilepsy, most likely of mesial temporal lobe origin. The commonest cause is hippocampal sclerosis which is readily identified on MRI. An EEG would also be useful, but the history is not suggestive of frontal lobe epilepsy.

Ophthalmology

Answer to Question 223

A

There are two well-defined, rounded, raised, choroidal lesions typical of metastases from carcinoma of the breast. These are more common than is clinically recognised because they often do not affect vision. Radiotherapy is an effective palliation, improving vision in a case such as this where the overall prognosis makes the risk of radiation-induced cataract and retinopathy irrelevant.

Answer to Question 224

D

There is a dense white opacity involving the disc margin from 2 to 8 o'clock, which also obscures the retinal vessels: this is due to myelinated nerve fibres. The upper edge of the disc is visible, well-defined and of normal appearance, excluding papilloedema and optic atrophy.

Answer to Question 225

B

There is proliferative retinopathy with obvious new vessels at the disc, a pre-retinal haemorrhage on the nasal side of the disc, and scars of panretinal photocoagulation. The macula appears healthy, without haemorrhages or hard exudates.

Answer to Question 226

B

Sarcoidosis is more common in Afro-Caribbean patients. A chest radiograph may show typical sarcoid changes to account for her chest symptoms. The presentation of a painful red eye, especially with photophobia, and treatment with frequent and potent topical corticosteroid together with pupillary dilatation, strongly suggests a slit-lamp diagnosis of acute iritis (anterior uveitis).

While rheumatoid arthritis may cause fatigue and joint pain, acute arthritis is a more typical presentation. Dry eye rarely presents so dramatically in one eye, and the treatment regime would be inappropriate for this. Iritis is not a common association. Wegener's granulomatosis could account for the non-specific systemic features, but uveitis is a much less common association than acute scleritis. Though topical corticosteroids might be used in scleritis, they are less appropriate, less likely to succeed, and dilating the pupil is unnecessary. Relapsing polychondritis is a contender as iritis may be associated, but there are no other specific features, such as swelling of the pinna or nasal cartilage, to suggest this very uncommon diagnosis in this case. Ankylosing spondylitis may be associated with acute iritis but multiple peripheral joint involvement is atypical and chest symptoms would not be expected.

Answer to Question 227

B

Her symptoms are typical of oedema within the central retina, affecting the fovea. Distortion and micropsia arise when the photoreceptors within the deeper layers of the retina become irregularly spaced. Such symptoms are typical of diabetic maculopathy, but not typical of proliferative retinopathy which is characteristically asymptomatic until an acute vitreous haemorrhage occurs.

Cataract occurs at an earlier age than usual in diabetes, but these symptoms are not typical. Retinal vein occlusion may present with foveal oedema but is less likely as a cause, especially in a relatively young woman without extra vascular risk factors. Oral hypoglycaemic medication does not cause foveal damage. Although transient blurring of vision may occur when the blood sugar is first brought under control, this is more typical of type 1 diabetes, in which normalisation is more rapid and more profound after using insulin for the first time.

Answer to Question 228

D

Cataract is common in renal transplant patients: risk factors include renal failure and long-term systemic corticosteroid medication. The symptoms are typical, as vision becomes worse in bright light when the pupil constricts, confining the light path to the central part of the lens where it is thickest and the typical steroid-induced cataract most pronounced.

Psychiatry

Answer to Question 229

E, H

It can be difficult to differentiate between depression and the sadness associated with an impending and untimely death. Thoughts of guilt and self-worthlessness are usually found in those who are depressed and it is unusual for those who are sad not to gain some enjoyment from some activities. Other questions should include those about suicidal thoughts.

Answer to Question 230

A

Acute stress disorder is a short-lived but severe disorder caused by an overwhelming, psychologically traumatic experience. The symptoms develop rapidly but tend to resolve within a matter of days. These include psychological symptoms, such as feeling numb and detached, dazed and disorientated, and physical symptoms, such as sweating, shakiness, palpitations and insomnia. Some patients will go on to develop post-traumatic stress disorder. If there is persistent denial that the event has occurred, the patient should be cautiously prompted to recall the facts.

A short course of a benzodiazepine tranquilliser and/or hypnotic may help severe agitation or insomnia.

Answer to Question 231

E

It was essential to check the ECG and pulse oximetry, but the clinical context and examination findings all point to the diagnosis of a panic attack, and – given that these tests gave normal results – it would be appropriate to explain the diagnosis to the patient and reassure accordingly. Psychological symptoms of an anxiety state include irritability, intolerance of noise, poor concentration/memory, fearfulness, apprehensiveness, restlessness and continuous worrying thoughts. Physical symptoms of an anxiety state include dry mouth, difficulty in swallowing, chest pain, shakiness, diarrhoea, urinary frequency, paraesthesiae and hot flushes. Physical signs of an anxiety state include tenseness, sweating, shaking, pallor, restlessness and sighing.

Answer to Question 232

B

High risk clinical factors for suicide include severe insomnia, self neglect, memory impairment, agitation, panic attacks, pessimism, despair, anhedonia and morbid guilt. Other factors predicting high risk are declared intent, preparation, past history of deliberate self harm (DSH), severe depression, schizophrenia and substance abuse, and the use of a potentially lethal method. However, patients are not experts in pharmacology, and taking a small overdose of a relatively safe drug (as in this case) does not mean that the suicide risk is necessarily low. For 10 years after an episode of DSH the risk of suicide is increased 30-fold over that expected: 1% of patients kill themselves in the year after an episode of DSH, and 20–25% of people who die by suicide have presented to hospital after episodes of DSH in the year before their death.

Answer to Question 233

A

In an Accident and Emergency department the suicidal patient who declines to be admitted for observation and treatment should be managed as follows: ensure that a member of staff stays with them at all times; call the duty psychiatrist; if they attempt to abscond before or during psychiatric assessment, the staff of the Accident and Emergency department have a duty under English Common Law to restrain the patient. If a patient who is already being nursed on medical, surgical or obstetric ward, or in a high dependency or intensive care unit, develops a mental illness (or has an exacerbation of a preexisting disorder), their physician or surgeon can authorise their compulsory detention for up to 72 hours under section 5(2) of the Mental Health Act.

Answer to Question 234

A

Depression is common in patients with advanced cancer (20–25% incidence) and can respond to treatment. Diagnosing depression with screening tools such as the Hospital Anxiety and Depression scale (HAD) or basic clinical interview should be within the capabilities of all doctors. In a clinic setting you should screen for depression, which includes listening to her concerns. If her feelings overwhelm her it is important to ask if she has thought about taking her own life. Studies suggest that patients do not often volunteer this but appreciate being asked, and it does not 'put ideas into their head'. Good communication with the primary care team about appropriate management, that might include antidepressants, is vital.

Endocrinology

Answer to Question 235

D

The appearances are typical of Turner's syndrome, with webbed neck and a wide carrying angle. The thoracotomy scar is a result of surgery to repair an atrial septal defect. The diagnosis is confirmed by finding a 45XO karyotype. The amenorrhoea is due to hypergonadotrophic hypogonadism with low / undetectable levels of oestradiol (E_2) and high levels of LH and FSH.

Answer to Question 236

B

Screening tests for Cushing's syndrome include (1) 24 hour urinary free cortisol estimation, (2) overnight dexamethasone suppression test, (3) low-dose dexamethasone suppression test, (4) loss of diurnal cortisol variation. Estimation of plasma ACTH level is important in determining whether Cushing's syndrome is ACTH-dependent (Cushing's disease due to pituitary adenoma, ectopic ACTH or rarely ectopic CRH secretion) or ACTH-independent (exogenous glucocorticoid, adrenal tumour, nodular adrenal hyperplasia), but is not appropriate for diagnosing whether or not Cushing's syndrome is present.

Answer to Question 237
D, H

Moderate to severe hypertension in a relatively young man in association with persistent hypokalaemia raises several possibilities. It may be due to essential hypertension in association with another cause for hypokalaemia such as diuretic therapy. However, rarer possibilities such as pheochromocytoma, primary hyperaldosteronism and Cushing's syndrome must be considered. In this case, suppressed plasma renin activity (PRA) in conjunction with significantly raised levels of aldosterone demonstrate that the normal feedback loop has broken down, and point to primary hyperaldosteronism as the most likely explanation. The findings are compatible with all different causes of primary hyperaldosteronism including Conn's syndrome (adenoma, ~65% of cases) and idiopathic hyperaldosteronism (bilateral adrenal zona glomerulosa hyperplasia, ~30%). In renal artery stenosis, PRA will also be high with high aldosterone levels, and in habitual excessive liquorice ingestion, both PRA and aldosterone levels will be low.

Answer to Question 238
C, H

The stress of diabetic ketoacidosis (DKA) itself can lead to a raised white blood cell count and amylase is also raised in this condition (perhaps salivary in origin) and so cannot be used as a reliable indicator of the presence or absence of pancreatitis in this circumstance. Bicarbonate therapy is not of benefit and is probably harmful in DKA when the pH is >6.9: no trials have been conducted on subjects presenting with pH lower than this. Total body potassium and phosphate are both depleted in DKA: plasma potassium concentration is raised because this intracellular cation is displaced from the intracellular compartment in acidotic conditions. DKA is primarily the result of unrestrained lipolysis and gluconeogenesis, augmented by the raised levels of counter-regulatory hormones (principally glucagon and catecholamines) found in this condition. It is lipolysis and unrestrained gluconeogenesis that lead to ketosis, and this is the process that needs to be reversed in order to improve acidosis. Remember, it is the acidosis that kills patients, not a high blood glucose reading. The low sodium concentration is partly due to electrolyte losses but is also partly artefactual. 3-hydroxybutyrate concentrations in plasma are usually two to three times those of acetoacetate, but in acidotic states this ratio is increased further.

Answer to Question 239
E, F

This man appears to have his hypertension and diabetes under good control and well within the targets. He has nephropathy with significant proteinuria and moderately advanced renal impairment. He is a smoker and has significantly raised cholesterol with reduced HDL and is running a high risk for ischaemic heart disease. He should stop smoking, try to maintain a healthy lifestyle with regular exercise and will benefit from seeing a dietician for appropriate advice regarding his lipid profile and weight (if overweight). He should be started on a statin in sufficient dose to lower his cholesterol to at least <5 mmol/l and may draw benefit from a regular low dose aspirin (if there are no contraindications). His renal impairment puts him at risk of lactic acidosis with metformin, which should be stopped.

Answer to Question 240
A

Hirsutism can occasionally be a sign of serious underlying pathology. If the history is of only six months, then this would increase the possibility that the woman may have an underlying virilising adrenal or ovarian tumour.

Answer to Question 241
C

The classical cause of primary hyperaldosteronism is a benign aldosterone-producing adenoma of the adrenal gland (Conn's syndrome). Other causes of primary hyperaldosteronism include idiopathic hyperaldosteronism associated with bilateral adrenal hyperplasia (the commonest cause), adrenal carcinoma and glucocorticoid remediable aldosteronism (GRA). Treatment with spironolactone is helpful in reducing the levels of mineralocorticoid, hence controlling blood pressure and restoring normokalaemia. Definitive and long-term treatments differ for each aetiology. Adrenalectomy is appropriate for Conn's adenoma and adrenal carcinoma. Long-term treatment with spironolactone or amiloride is the treatment of choice in idiopathic hyperaldosteronism associated with bilateral adrenal hyperplasia. Glucocorticoids are useful in patients with GRA, which is a very rare autosomal dominant disorder where the synthesis of mineralocorticoids becomes adrenocorticotropic hormone (ACTH) dependent and therapy with glucocorticoid reduces ACTH levels through a negative feedback mechanism leading to a reduction in ACTH-dependent mineralocorticoid production.

Answer to Question 242

E

The testes are normally under control from the pituitary, but in this case it appears from the limited information given that testosterone production is occurring independently of the pituitary, indeed the level is sufficient to have suppressed gonadotrophin production. Possible causes are a testosterone-producing (or hCG-producing) tumour (testicular, adrenal or elsewhere), exogenous testosterone administration, or testosterone hyperproduction as a side effect of a block in glucocorticoid synthesis (due to a variant of congenital adrenal hyperplasia, CAH). Priorities should be testicular examination and a careful clinical and biochemical search for an androgen-secreting tumour and questioning about self-administration of testosterone or an analogue. If CAH is to be sought, the level of 17-hydroxyprogesterone (17-OHP) at 09.00 h is most informative as production is entrained to ACTH levels. A short synacthen test should also be performed with both 17-OHP and cortisol measurements if the clinical suspicion remains.

Answer to Question 243

B

Patients with Cushing's syndrome may have different presentations and features depending upon the cause. Most patients will have features that are more or less typical of Cushing's, but those with ectopic ACTH from a malignant tumour or a malignant adrenal tumour may present rapidly with weight loss, hypertension, hypokalaemia, obvious tumour and features of its spread, and not much in the way of Cushingoid features. Patients with an adrenal adenoma do not have features of hyperandrogenaemia like hirsutism because benign adrenal tumours produce cortisol but not androgens. Absence of hirsutism and virilisation in a patient with other features of Cushing's syndrome favours adrenal adenoma but needs further investigation. A normal MRI scan of the pituitary does not differentiate between different non-pituitary dependent causes of Cushing's syndrome.

Answer to Question 244

C

It is quite obvious from his drug history, biochemical profile and blood pressure that the patient is being over treated with fludrocortisone. His recent cortisol day profile reflects satisfactory replacement with glucocorticoids. Treating him with antihypertensives may help but does not make sense. If his blood pressure remains high despite reduction of fludrocortisone dosage, he may then need antihypertensives.

Answer to Question 245

D

Primary hyperaldosteronism is an important cause of hypertenison in the young to middle aged. Most cases are caused by bilateral adrenal hyperplasia. If potassium depletion is severe then polydipsia, polyuria, paraesthesiae and alkalosis may occur. Headaches are common. Retinopathy is mild and retinal haemorrhages are rarely seen.

Answer to Question 246

B

Patients managed by diet alone need not notify the Driver and Vehicle Licensing Agency (DVLA) unless they develop relevant disabilities (such as eye problems) or they need drug treatment for their diabetes. Patients managed with oral hypoglycaemic agents can retain their licence up to the age of 70 years unless they develop relevant disabilities or need insulin treatment for their diabetes. Patients managed on insulin must demonstrate satisfactory control, recognise warning symptoms of hypoglycaemia and meet required visual standards. They will be given a one, two or three-year licence. Patients with insulin-treated gestational diabetes must notify the DVLA but may retain their licence if they have good control. Patients with diabetes and eyesight complications have the same rules as non-diabetic drivers.

Answer to Question 247

C

The man clearly has poorly controlled diabetes. It is likely that he has diabetic retinopathy and very important to exclude sight-threatening maculopathy or proliferative retinopathy. His blurred vision may be due to poor glycaemic control but it is vital to perform fundoscopy and exclude any retinopathy that requires urgent ophthalmological attention.

The patient has dipsticks positive proteinuria, hence estimation of urinary albumin:creatinine ratio is pointless. Estimation of 24-hour urinary protein excretion would be appropriate to quantify the proteinuria and ultrasound of renal tract to see the size of kidneys and to exclude obstructive uropathy may also be justified. A radiograph of his foot and possibly some other imaging will also be needed to assess this problem. However, preservation of his sight from imminent threats must be the highest priority.

Answer to Question 248

D

Maculopathy is the commonest threat to vision in type 2 diabetes. It typically produces loss of central vision and if discovered or suspected requires urgent referral to an ophthalmologist. The 3-year risk of severe visual loss in maculopathy is reduced by over 50% with photocoagulation: macular grid laser therapy is usually used. Both glycaemia and hypertension should be as well controlled as possible. Circinate exudates occur around areas of microvascular leakage and should therefore lead to the suspicion of macular ischaemia.

Answer to Question 249

C

This woman appears to have cranial diabetes insipidus secondary to metastatic disease from her breast cancer. Her investigations are not complete, but DDAVP in the form of nasal spray or subcutaneous injections appears to be the most suitable treatment, with the patient allowed to drink according to her thirst. Intravenous 5% dextrose will be appropriate if the patient is unable to drink and the serum sodium concentration is rising.

Hydrochlorothiazide may be used to treat nephrogenic diabetes insipidus. Demeclocycline and lithium carbonate induce nephrogenic diabetes insipidus and may be used to treat the syndrome of inappropriate antidiuresis (SIADH).

Nephrology

Answer to Question 250

E

Figure 34 shows a 'trash foot' with the appearance of livido reticularis resulting from cutaneous ischaemia associated with distal embolisation. In the context of a ruptured abdominal aortic aneurysm this man would clearly be at risk of acute tubular necrosis (and perhaps acute cortical necrosis), but the condition suggested by the appearance of his foot is cholesterol embolisation. It is most unlikely that renal biopsy would be performed in this case, but the appearance of cholesterol clefts within renal vessels is diagnostic. There is no effective treatment for this condition and the prognosis for renal recovery is poor.

Answer to Question 251

A

The appearances are typical of medullary sponge kidney, which is a common cause of medullary nephrocalcinosis as shown in Figure 35. The cause of this condition is unknown, but some cases are familial. The most important aspect of treatment is to encourage the patient to drink enough to maintain a urinary volume of at least 2 litres/day, which is the best way to prevent recurrent stone formation.

Answer to Question 252

D, F

There are a number of possible causes of renal disease in rheumatoid arthritis. Chronic inflammation can result in AA amyloidosis. Gold and penicillamine used in treatment can cause a membranous nephropathy. Non-steroidal anti-inflammatory drugs can cause a fall in glomerular filtration rate, an interstitial nephritis and minimal change nephropathy. Patients with rheumatoid arthritis can develop aggressive vasculitis resulting in rapidly progressive glomerulonephritis. In this case the heavy proteinuria and renal impairment would fit with either a membranous nephropathy or AA amyloid.

Answer to Question 253

C, F

This is a typical presentation of systemic amyloidosis. It is likely that the patient has the AL (immunocyte-related) form of the condition, based on the presence of the paraprotein and the low CRP. A renal biopsy is required to establish the cause of the nephrotic syndrome: amyloidosis is likely, but other primary glomerular disease cannot be confidently excluded without histology. A bone marrow aspirate and trephine are needed because some degree of plasma cell dyscrasia is likely, and if there is frank myeloma treatment is indicated. Even if there is no frank myeloma, some treatment, e.g. prednisolone and melphalan, may be warranted since untreated amyloid tends to progress rapidly, and AL-amyloid can lead to rapid cardiac and renal decompensation.

Answer to Question 254

D

The patient has an inappropriately high level of PTH for her serum calcium level, but the reduced urine calcium excretion suggests that she has familial hypocalcuric hypercalcaemia (FHH) due to a mutation in the calcium receptor. Urinary calcium excretion is increased in patients with hyperparathyroidism in the absence of vitamin D deficiency but is low in patients with FHH, as is the case here. The urinary calcium to creatinine ratio is useful in identifying the 2–5% of patients who have FHH and who might otherwise be thought to have a parathyroid adenoma. Here this diagnosis is also supported by the probable family history.

Answer to Question 255

E

Liddle's syndrome is caused by a mutation in the sodium channel (ENaC) in the distal nephron. The mutation keeps the channel open, which has a similar effect to a raised aldosterone level, including increased potassium excretion leading to hypokalaemia. Aldosterone levels are not raised and may be lowered as a result of feedback from sodium and water retention. The condition is sometimes called pseudohyperaldosteronism.

Answer to Question 256

D

Von Hippel Lindau disease is an autosomal dominant condition. Affected individuals may have any of the following: renal cysts; clear cell renal cell carcinoma (CCRCC); retinal angiomas; central nervous system haemangioblastoma; phaeochromocytoma. Another manifestation is endolymphatic sac tumours, causing deafness. Below 3 cm, solid lesions in the kidneys can be monitored, but above this size usual practice would be to remove them. Hypertension suggests this patient may have a phaeochromocytoma.

Answer to Question 257

B

Adult polycystic kidney disease (APKD) is the most common inherited renal disease leading to end-stage renal failure, accounting for about 4% of those receiving renal replacement therapy. There are two known loci: PKD1 on chromosome 16 accounts for 85% of cases and PKD2 on chromosome 4 for 10%. Presentation is with ab-

dominal pain, haematuria, hypertension, urinary tract infection, incidental discovery of an abdominal mass, or as a result of family screening (or serendipitous imaging of the kidneys, e.g. by ultrasound examination ordered for another purpose).

Answer to Question 258

A

The diagnosis is minimal change glomerulonephritis, also known as minimal change nephropathy, minimal change disease, lipoid nephrosis and idiopathic nephrotic syndrome. Standard initial therapy is with corticosteroids, typically prednisolone at a dose of about 1 mg/kg/day, which introduces remission in around 80% of patients. Supportive therapies are also given, diuretics to clear oedema will clearly be appropriate in this case, and some nephrologists would prescribe warfarin to reduce risk of thromboembolism and a statin to reduce hypercholesterolaemia, although many would elect to see whether or not the patient went into a rapid remission that would render these agents unnecessary. Ciclosporin is useful as a steroid-sparing agent in patients who frequently relapse but would not be used as initial treatment.

Answer to Question 259

E

This man has nephritic syndrome, which is the combination of hypertension, oedema, proteinuria and renal impairment. Focal segmental glomerulosclerosis typically presents with the nephrotic syndrome. In post infectious glomerulonephritis, which otherwise would fit with this presentation, the infection is usually clinically apparent, hence the most likely diagnosis is mesangiocapillary glomerulonephritis. Hypocomplementaemia is typical of this condition.

Answer to Question 260

A

Mixed essential cryoglobulinaemia will often present with palpable purpura on the legs and nephritis, but is an uncommon disease of older patients. If the man did not have a rash, then IgA nephropathy would be the most probable cause of his urinary findings.

Answer to Question 261

B

There is an association between severe obesity and focal segmental glomerulosclerosis, which is the most likely diagnosis in this case.

Answer to Question 262

B

In any patient with a history of chronic progressive worsening of symptoms and renal impairment it is important to consider systemic vasculitis as a possible cause. In this case the rash and sinusitis are further pointers. Often a patient with systemic vasculitis will have a long history of indolent disease but will then present late with severe aggressive disease. Sinusitis suggests involvement of the nasal tract and sinuses in Wegener's granulomatosis. Useful immunological tests include assays for antineutrophil cytoplasmic antibodies (ANCA) and direct assays for antibodies against the ANCA antigens myeloperoxidase and proteinase 3.

Answer to Question 263

A

Diabetic nephropathy is a microvascular complication and rarely occurs without other evidence of microvascular disease such as retinopathy. It is often associated with suboptimal glycaemic control and proteinuria. Renal size is preserved, but following the development of microalbuminuria the disease may progress with alarming rapidity.

Answer to Question 264

C

Systemic lupus erythematosus (SLE) is a common condition and the prevalence is higher in women than men and in black people than white. Typical features include skin rashes, neurological or psychiatric abnormalities, and renal disease. Elevation of the ESR with a normal CRP is typical of SLE.

Rheumatology and Clinical Immunology

Answer to Question 265

C

With this history, the diagnosis is meningococcal septicaemia. This is a fulminant disease, delay of a few hours can be fatal, and immediate treatment with intravenous benzylpenicillin or cefotaxime should be given.

Meningococcal septicaemia can affect a normal host, but patients with a deficiency of a terminal complement component are particularly susceptible. This can most easily be detected by measuring the CH50 or CH100, which tests the ability of the complement in the patient's serum to lyse erythrocytes by the classical complement pathway. If any complement component (C1-9) is missing, lysis will not occur.

Answer to Question 266

D

The hand is critically ischaemic with impending gangrene. The pattern of immunofluorescence is typical of an anticentromere antibody, with multiple fine dots due to staining of the kinetochores of the 23 pairs of chromosomes. In this clinical context, anticentromere antibodies are reliable markers of the CREST syndrome (Calcinosis, Raynaud's, Esophageal dysfunction, Sclerodactyly, Telangiectasia), also known as limited cutaneous systemic sclerosis.

Answer to Question 267

A

The kidney biopsy shows striking linear deposits of IgG along the glomerular basement membrane (GBM), indicating the presence of anti-GBM antibodies diagnostic (in this clinical context) of Goodpasture's disease.

Answer to Question 268

B, E

Swelling of the distal interphalangeal joints really only occurs in nodal osteoarthritis and one of the forms of psoriatic arthritis, which is usually easily distinguished by nail involvement (not present in this case).

Involvement of the base of the thumb is also pathognomonic of nodal osteoarthritis, giving the thumb base a characteristically square appearance.

Answer to Question 269

C, G

The most likely cause of these symptoms is rheumatoid arthritis, but SLE requires careful consideration.

Rheumatoid arthritis can present as an acute monoarthritis, an acute polyarthritis, a subacute insidious polyarthritis, or with a polymyalgic presentation (particularly in the elderly, when it needs to be differentiated from polymyalgia rheumatica).

Remember that acute synovitis in early rheumatoid arthritis is associated with very little fixed joint deformity and no extra-articular features. This contrasts with the deforming arthritis that is characteristic of chronic disease.

Answer to Question 270

B

It would be important to exclude septic arthritis by microscopy and culture of fluid aspirated from the knee, but this is not the commonest cause of an acute monoarthritis.

The differential diagnosis is influenced by age. Crystal arthritis is the most common cause in elderly people, whereas reactive arthritis tends to occur in sexually active young adults.

Calcium pyrophosphate deposition disease, often known as pseudogout, can often present with striking fever and systemic illness. Treatment is with NSAIDs or intra-articular steroid injection, once sepsis has been excluded.

Answer to Question 271

A, I

The most likely cause of a vertebral crush factor in a woman of this age is obviously osteoporosis, but local vertebral pathology – in particular secondary tumours or myeloma – would need to be considered.

It is most likely that the cause of osteoporosis would be 'postmenopausal' in this woman, but many medical factors influence the likelihood of this condition.

The following tests should be considered in a patient presenting with an osteoporotic fracture (although not all need to be performed in all cases): full blood count, renal/liver/bone chemistry, immunoglobulins and serum/urine electrophoresis (to exclude myeloma), thyroid function, testosterone (in men), investigations for Cushing's syndrome.

Answer to Question 272

B, E

The important complications of systemic sclerosis to consider are interstitial lung disease, pulmonary hypertension and cardiac disease (usually myocardial, sometimes pericardial). Pulmonary emboli are fairly common in the context of connective tissue disease, especially when cardiolipin antibodies are present. Diaphragmatic weakness can occur, due to myopathy, but would not produce marked reduction in gas transfer.

Answer to Question 273

F, H

The diagnosis is polymyalgia rheumatica. This will usually respond dramatically to small doses of prednisolone, which will be required for an average duration of 12–18 months before the disease goes into remission. The major side effect of such low doses of steroid is osteoporosis and prophylaxis will usually be required.

Answer to Question 274

A

Active SLE and tuberculosis are both associated with leukopenia. Low titre antinuclear antibodies (in the absence of DNA or ENA), antineutrophil cytoplasmic antibodies (ANCA) and anticardiolipin antibodies are non-specific and are commonly found in the presence of infection.

Answer to Question 275

B

Henoch–Schönlein purpura (HSP) is characterised by the tissue deposition of IgA-containing immune complexes. The pathogenesis of this disorder appears similar to that of IgA nephropathy, which is associated with identical histologic findings in the kidney.

HSP is commoner in children than in adults. Many cases follow an upper respiratory tract infection, suggesting that the precipitating antigen may be infectious. The clinical manifestations include a classic tetrad of rash, arthralgias, abdominal pain, and renal disease that can occur in any order and at any time over a period of several days to several weeks. The rash is typically purpuric and distributed symmetrically over the lower legs and arms: clotting studies are normal.

Answer to Question 276

E

The lack of constitutional symptoms, normal inflammatory markers and normal examination, apart from evidence of tender points, make an inflammatory rheumatological disease unlikely. The presence of tender points, history of muscle pain and sleep disturbance are suggestive of fibromyalgia – a non-inflammatory pain disorder.

Answer to Question 277

C

Arthritis with predominant involvement of the distal interphalangeal joint occurs most often in generalised osteoarthritis and psoriatic arthritis. The fact that this patient is relatively young and has a raised ESR indicates an underlying inflammatory disease is the most likely cause of her symptoms, hence psoriatic arthritis is the most likely diagnosis in this case. Examination of the skin and nails for psoriasis is very important in confirming the diagnosis. The scalp hairline, the naval and the palms are areas often involved in psoriasis but easily missed.

Rheumatoid arthritis and SLE are known to affect the proximal interphalangeal (PIPs) and the metacarpophalangeal (MCPs) joints. Chronic gouty arthritis might involve the DIPs, but more often it involves the MCPs and PIPs in asymmetrical fashion with or without tophus formation.

Answer to Question 278

A

Pseudogout occurs when there are acute attacks of CPPD crystal-induced synovitis, which clinically resembles acute gout caused by urate crystals. However, most patients with CPPD crystal deposition in their joints never experience such episodes. A variety of metabolic and endocrine disorders are associated with CPPD crystal deposition, including diabetes mellitus, haemochromatosis, Wilson's disease, hypothyroidism, hyperparathyroidism, hypomagnesaemia and hypophosphatasia.

Answer to Question 279

E

This patient has acute gout, probably diuretic-induced. Intra-articular corticosteroids are safe and highly efficacious in this situation, once sepsis is excluded.

Allopurinol has no role in the acute treatment of gout. Colchicine at these doses is very poorly tolerated due to GI toxicity. Non-steroidals are very likely to precipitate deterioration in renal function and may also exacerbate heart failure.

Answer to Question 280

D

About 25% of patients with rheumatoid arthritis (RA) have ocular manifestations, including keratoconjunctivitis sicca, scleritis, episcleritis, keratitis, peripheral corneal ulceration and other less common entities such as choroiditis, retinal vasculitis, episcleral nodules, retinal detachments and macular oedema.

Keratoconjunctivitis sicca, or dry eye syndrome, presents as 'gritty eyes' and is the most common ocular manifestation of RA (prevalence 15–25 %).

Answer to Question 281

E

Paget's disease is a focal disorder of bone remodelling characterised by an increase in the number and size of osteoclasts in affected skeletal sites, whilst the rest of the skeleton is spared. It can affect any bone, but the axial skeleton, particularly the pelvis, is usual. In most cases at least two bones are affected. Hearing loss through compression of the 8th nerve occurs in 30–40% of patients. Other causes of hearing loss include pagetic involvement of the middle ear ossicles, but this is relatively rare.

Unlike osteoarthritis, pagetic bone pain usually increases with rest, on weight bearing, when the limbs are warmed, and at night, but 70% or so of patients with Paget's disease have no symptoms, the diagnosis being found incidentally by radiographs and laboratory investigations.

Answer to Question 282

D

Aspiration of the knee with microscopy to look for pus cells / organisms in the case of septic arthritis and crystals in the case of gout or pseudogout is the most useful investigation. Blood cultures may yield an organism. A radiograph would be useful as a baseline but is unlikely to show acute changes and is not the top priority. Uric acid levels may not be elevated in an acute episode of gout. A raised CRP is non-specific, but can be used to monitor the effectiveness of treatment.

Index